Radiotherapy in Skin Cancer

Kurian Jones Joseph • Michael J. Veness
Elizabeth Barnes • Agata Rembielak
Editors

Radiotherapy in Skin Cancer

A Practical Guide on Indications and Techniques

Springer

Editors
Kurian Jones Joseph
Division of Radiation Oncology, Cross Cancer Institute
University of Alberta
Edmonton, AB, Canada

Elizabeth Barnes
Department of Radiation Oncology, Odette Cancer Centre
University of Toronto
Toronto, ON, Canada

Michael J. Veness
Department of Radiation Oncology
Westmead Hospital, University of Sydney
Westmead, NSW, Australia

Agata Rembielak
Department of Clinical Oncology
The Christie NHS Foundation Trust
Manchester, UK

Division of Cancer Sciences
School of Medical Sciences
Faculty of Biology, Medicine and Health
The University of Manchester
Manchester, UK

ISBN 978-3-031-44315-2 ISBN 978-3-031-44316-9 (eBook)
https://doi.org/10.1007/978-3-031-44316-9

This Springer imprint is published by the registered company Springer Nature Switzerland AG
The registered company address is: Gewerbestrasse 11, 6330 Cham, Switzerland

Paper in this product is recyclable.

Foreword

I am delighted to present this exceptional handbook on radiotherapy indications and techniques for skin cancer. Skin cancer is one of the most prevalent types of cancer, with a global incidence that continues to escalate. Radiotherapy is a valuable treatment modality for skin cancer, offering a noninvasive and highly effective approach for both early and advanced stages of the disease.

The editorial team comprises Kurian Joseph, Michael Veness, Elizabeth Barnes, and Agata Rembielak who are eminent oncologists, whose extensive knowledge and expertise in the field of skin cancer have culminated in this remarkable compendium. The handbook provides an outstanding overview of skin cancer, including its various types and the stages where radiotherapy is deemed appropriate.

The handbook is also replete with an array of techniques of radiotherapy that are deployed in skin cancer treatment, ranging from superficial radiation therapy to brachytherapy and electron beam therapy. Each technique is meticulously explained, with detailed descriptions of the equipment and procedures involved.

Moreover, it underscores important considerations such as patient selection, treatment planning, and follow-up care. The authors have provided practical guidance on how to manage acute and late radiation toxicities, as well as strategies for optimizing treatment outcomes.

This handbook will be a precious resource for radiation oncologists, dermatologists, and other healthcare professionals, who are committed to the care of patients with skin cancer. My hope is that it will contribute significantly to optimizing radiotherapy in the management of skin cancer, ultimately enhancing patient outcomes and their quality of life.

Department of Radiation Oncology
Northwest Community Hospital
Arlington Heights, IL, USA

Najeeb Mohideen, MD,FRCR,FASTRO,FACR

Preface

In this first edition of our book, "Radiotherapy in Skin Cancer: Indications and Techniques—A Practical Guide," we have attempted to succinctly detail the indications and radiotherapy treatment techniques for the management of common skin cancers.

Radiotherapy plays a key role in skin cancer management. The treatment of skin cancer using radiotherapy is becoming increasingly complex with the introduction of modern radiotherapy techniques, such as IMRT/VMAT and imaging-based treatment planning. This book provides essential and updated information on the pathology of skin cancer, the AJCC/UICC staging systems, as well as the indications for and the various radiotherapy treatment techniques routinely used in the management of common skin cancers often seen in routine clinical practice and based on current evidence.

We are grateful to all the chapter authors, many of whom are international experts in their respective fields, for their valuable contributions.

We believe that this book will serve as a practical reference handbook for use in the day-to-day clinical practice for professionals involved in skin cancer management, especially radiation oncologists, dermatologists, surgeons, radiation therapists, and nurses including those who are in training.

Finally, we express our gratitude for the staff at "Springer Nature" group, especially Michelle Tam and Rekha Muthusamy, for their help and continued support in undertaking this project.

Edmonton, AB, Canada — Kurian Jones Joseph
Westmead, NSW, Australia — Michael J. Veness
Toronto, ON, Canada — Elizabeth Barnes(Toni)
Manchester, UK — Agata Rembielak

Contents

Editors and Contributors

About the Editors

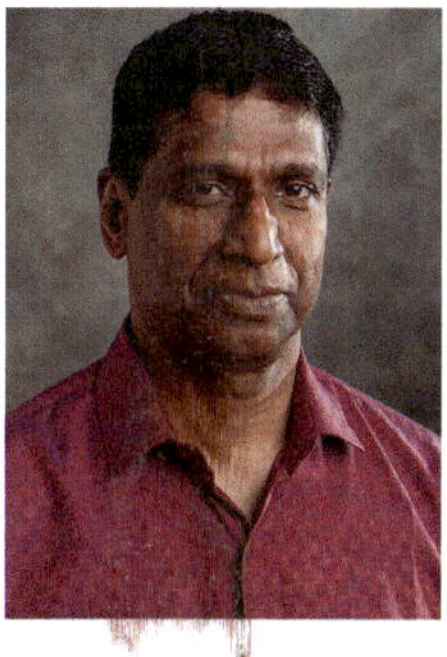

Kurian Jones Joseph is currently Professor at the Department of Oncology, University of Alberta, and is a senior radiation oncologist at the Cross Cancer Institute, Edmonton, Alberta, Canada.Dr. Joseph completed his undergraduate medical training at Calicut Medical College, India, and did his radiation oncology specialty training at the Regional Cancer Centre, Trivandrum, India, and at the Faculty of Radiology of the Royal College of Surgeons in Ireland. His primary area of interest is cutaneous malignancies. He has authored several peer-reviewed, national and international publications.

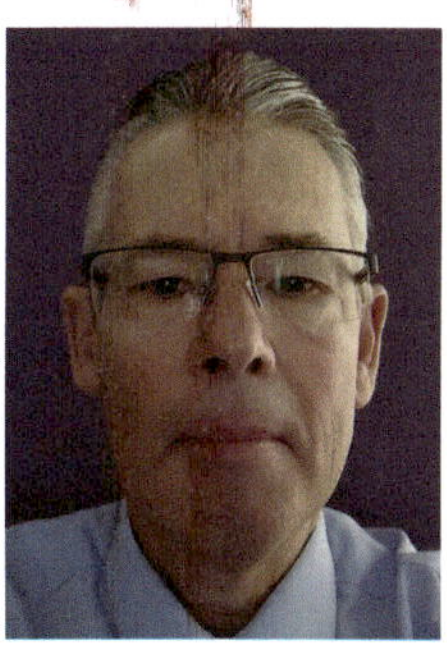

Michael J. Veness has been a full-time staff specialist in radiation oncology at Westmead Hospital, Sydney, since 1998. His clinical practice predominantly involves managing patients with mucosal and cutaneous malignancies of the head and neck. He has had a longstanding clinical research focus on the important and beneficial role of radiotherapy in treating patients with non-melanoma skin cancer and specifically in patients diagnosed with Merkel cell carcinoma (primary cutaneous neuroendocrine malignancy) and high-risk cutaneous squamous cell carcinomas (especially those with metastatic nodes). In addition to a master's degree in clinical epidemiology, he has been awarded MDs by published work (detailing the role of radiotherapy in both Merkel cell carcinoma and metastatic nodal SCC, respectively) from both the University of NSW and the University of Sydney and has published widely, both locally and internationally, over 160 peer-reviewed publications and book chapters on various skin cancer-related topics and is a clinical professor with the Sydney Medical School, University of Sydney. He is considered an international expert in this area and believes strongly in educating and informing clinicians managing patients with skin cancer of the often-underappreciated benefits, which in some cases can be lifesaving, to utilizing radiotherapy, be that definitive (i.e., radical), adjuvant (i.e., post-op), or palliative radiotherapy.

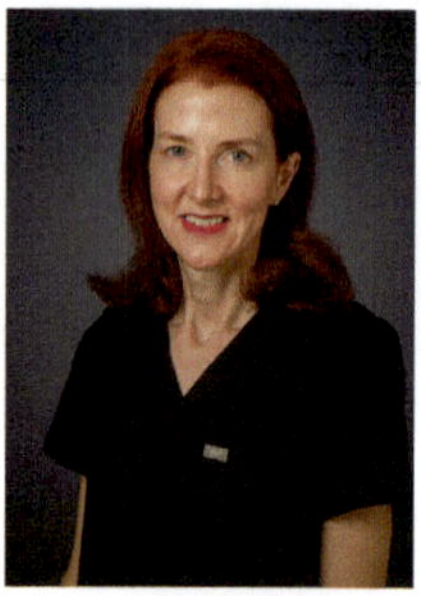

Elizabeth A. Barnes, MD, FRCPC (C) is a radiation oncologist at the Odette Cancer Centre and Associate Professor in the Department of Radiation Oncology, University of Toronto, Canada. Her clinical and research areas of interest are skin and gynecologic cancer.

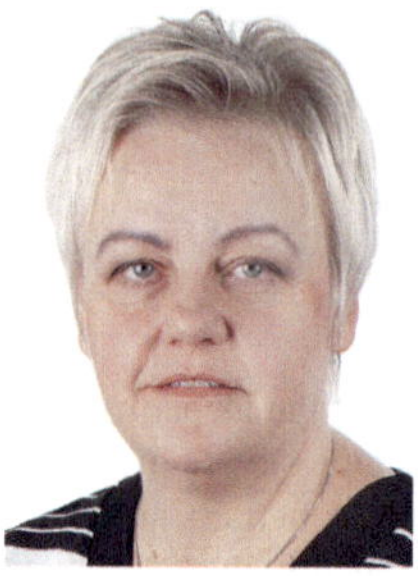

Agata Rembielak graduated in medicine and medical physics in Poland. She then enrolled in specialist training in radiation oncology in Poland and undertook clinical research fellowships in Australia, Canada, and the UK. She holds research degrees, MD and PhD, in both medical sciences and oncology. She has also been a keen medical educator, holding an MA in medical education.She works as a Clinical Oncology Consultant at the Christie Hospital in Manchester and has been appointed a MAHSC Chair at the University of Manchester. Her research interests include non-melanoma skin cancer, particularly the role of radiotherapy and brachytherapy in skin cancer management, palliative radiotherapy, and geriatric oncology. Within ESTRO, she is a director of the course "Multidisciplinary management of non-melanoma skin cancer" and leads the Skin and Soft Tissue Focus Group. She chairs the SIOG Task Force on non-melanoma skin cancer in older adults. Dr. Rembielak co-authored UK BAD guidelines on skin SCC and GEC-ESTRO guidelines on skin brachytherapy.

Contributors

Aswin George Abraham, MD, D.Phil Division of Radiation Oncology, Cross Cancer Institute, & Department of Oncology, University of Alberta, Edmonton, Canada

Elizabeth A. Barnes, MD, FRCPC Odette Cancer Centre, University of Toronto, Toronto, ON, Canada

Karen Pat-Ming Chu, MD FRCPC Department of Oncology, University of Alberta, Edmonton, AB, Canada

Division of Radiation Oncology, Cross Cancer Institute, Edmonton, AB, Canada

Arun Elangovan, MD Division of Radiation Oncology, Cross Cancer Institute, Edmonton, AB, Canada

Gerald B. Fogarty, BSc, MBBS, PhD, FRANZCR The Icon Cancer Centre, Sydney, NSW, Australia

University of Technology, Sydney, NSW, Australia

Angela M. Hong, MBBS, MMed PhD FRANZCR Melanoma Institute Australia, Faculty of Medicine and Health, University of Sydney, Sydney, NSW, Australia

Kurian Jones Joseph, MBBS, FFRRCSI,FRCR,FRCPC Division of Radiation Oncology, Cross Cancer Institute, Edmonton, AB, Canada

Department of Oncology, University of Alberta, Edmonton, AB, Canada

Michael E. Kasper, MD, FACRO Department of Radiation Oncology Lynn Cancer Institute, Boca Raton Regional Hospital, Boca Raton, FL, USA

Baptist Health Medical Group North, South Florida, USA

Beena Kunheri, MBBS, DNB, MNAMS, FRCR Hamad Medical Corporation, National Center for Cancer Care and Research (NCCCR), Doha, Qatar

Winkle Kwan, MD, FRCPC Division of Radiation Oncology, Department of Surgery, Faculty of Medicine, University of British Columbia, Vancouver, BC, Canada

Muhammad N. Mahmood, MD, FCAP Department of Laboratory Medicine & Pathology, University of Alberta Hospital, Edmonton, AB, Canada

Geetha Menon, PhD, FCCPM Department of Oncology, University of Alberta, Edmonton, AB, Canada

Department of Medical Physics, Cross Cancer Institute, Edmonton, AB, Canada

Romaana Mir, MBChB, MSc, MRCP, FRCR, MD(Res) Mount Vernon Cancer Centre, Northwood, UK

The Univeristy of Manchester, Manchester, UK

Sandro V. Porceddu, BSc, MBBS (Hons), FRANZCR, MD Faculty of Medicine, University of QLD, Brisbane, QLD, Australia

Peter MacCallum Cancer Centre, Melbourne, VIC, Australia

Department of Radiology, Faculty of Medicine, University of Melbourne, Melbourne, VIC, Australia

Agata Rembielak, MD, PhD, MA (Clin Ed), FRCR Department of Clinical Oncology, The Christie NHS Foundation Trust, Manchester, UK

Division of Cancer Sciences, School of Medical Sciences, Faculty of Biology, Medicine and Health, The University of Manchester, Manchester, UK

Hina Saeed, MD Department of Radiation Oncology, Lynn Cancer Institute, Boca Raton Regional Hospital, Baptist Health South Florida, Boca Raton, FL, USA

Justin Smith, MBBS (Hons), MPH Radiation Oncology Department, Princess Alexandra Hospital, Brisbane, QLD, Australia

Faculty of Medicine, University of QLD, Brisbane, QLD, Australia

College of Medicine and Dentistry, James Cook University, Townsville, QLD, Australia

Aoife Jones Thachuthara, MBBCh BAO (Hons) Department of Medicine, Beaumont Hospital, Dublin, Ireland

May N. Tsao, MD, FRCPC Odette Cancer Centre, University of Toronto, Toronto, ON, Canada

Michael. J. Veness, MD, FRANZCR Department of Radiation Oncology, Crown Princess Mary Cancer Centre, Westmead Hospital, Sydney, NSW, Australia

Edward Yu, MDCM, PhD, FRCPC Department of Oncology and Medical Biophysics, Western University, London, ON, Canada

Part I
General Principles of Skin Radiotherapy

Chapter 1
Classification and Pathology of Common Cutaneous Malignancies

Muhammad N. Mahmood

Introduction

Malignancies of the skin are among the most common health issues associated with a considerable burden on healthcare worldwide. Non-melanoma skin cancers (NMSCs) and melanoma significantly impact health services and have substantial public health significance. Ultraviolet (UV) radiation exposure plays a significant role in their development, as most neoplasms develop on chronically sun-exposed sites. Basal cell carcinoma (BCC) and squamous cell carcinoma (SCC) are the most frequent malignant neoplasms, and melanoma is one of the fastest-growing malignancies in the fair-skinned population. Melanoma accounts for about 75% of cutaneous malignancy-related deaths in the United States.

Malignancies of the skin comprise a broad range of numerous lesions and conditions. They are classified under six categories: epidermal tumor, cutaneous melanoma, malignant appendageal tumor, primary cutaneous lymphoma, and malignant cutaneous soft tissue tumor (Table 1.1) [1, 2]. The spectrum is broad and complex, with each category containing further subgroups and types. However, in everyday clinical practice, the commonly encountered malignancies include NMSCs (e.g., BCC, SCC, Merkel cell carcinoma) and melanoma.

M. N. Mahmood (✉)
Department of Laboratory Medicine & Pathology,
University of Alberta Hospital, Edmonton, AB, Canada
e-mail: muhammad.mahmood@albertaprecisionlabs.ca

K. J. Joseph et al. (eds.), *Radiotherapy in Skin Cancer*,
https://doi.org/10.1007/978-3-031-44316-9_1

Table 1.1 Classification of cutaneous malignancies

Epidermal tumors/carcinomas	Cutaneous melanomas	Malignant appendageal tumors	Primary cutaneous lymphomas	Malignant cutaneous soft tissue tumors/sarcomas
Basal cell carcinoma – Superficial BCC – Nodular BCC – Fibroepithelial BCC – Pigmented BCC – Infundibulocystic BCC – Micronodular BCC – Infiltrating BCC – Sclerosing/morpheaform BCC – Basosquamous carcinoma – BCC with sarcomatoid differentiation **Squamous cell carcinoma** – Keratoacanthomatous SCC – Verrucous SCC – Acantholytic SCC – Spindle cell SCC – Adenosquamous carcinoma – Clear-cell SCC – SCC, NOS **Merkel cell carcinoma**	Low-CSD melanoma • Superficial spreading melanoma High-CSD melanoma • Lentigo maligna melanoma • Desmoplastic melanoma (pure and mixed) Nodular melanoma Acral melanoma Nevoid melanoma Spitz melanoma Melanoma arising in a blue nevus Melanoma arising in a giant congenital nevus Melanoma, NOS	**Eccrine and apocrine differentiation** – Microcystic adnexal carcinoma – Porocarcinoma – Hidradenocarcinoma – Digital papillary adenocarcinoma – Eccrine ductal carcinoma – Squamoid eccrine ductal carcinoma – Malignant mixed tumor – Malignant neoplasms arising from spiradenoma or cylindroma – Adenoid cystic carcinoma – Apocrine carcinoma – Syringocystadenocarcinoma papilliferum – Mucinous carcinoma – Endocrine mucin-producing sweat duct carcinoma – Signet-ring cell/histiocytoid carcinoma **Follicular differentiation** – Pilomatrical carcinoma – Proliferating trichilemmal tumor – Trichilemmal carcinoma – Trichoblastic carcinoma/carcinosarcoma **Sebaceous differentiation** – Sebaceous carcinoma (ocular and extraocular) **Site-specific tumors** – Mammary Paget's disease – Extramammary Paget's disease	**Cutaneous T-cell lymphomas** • Mycosis fungoides • MF variants: – Folliculotropic MF – Pagetoid reticulosis – Granulomatous slack skin • Sézary syndrome • Primary cutaneous CD30-positive LPD – Primary cutaneous anaplastic large-cell lymphoma – Lymphomatoid papulosis • Adult T-cell leukemia/ lymphoma • Subcutaneous panniculitis-like T-cell lymphoma • Extranodal NK/T-cell lymphoma, nasal type • Primary cutaneous gamma-delta T-cell lymphoma • Primary cutaneous CD4+ small/ medium T-cell LPD • Primary cutaneous peripheral T-cell lymphoma, NOS **Cutaneous B-cell lymphomas** – Primary cutaneous marginal zone lymphoma – Primary cutaneous follicle center lymphoma – Primary cutaneous diffuse large B-cell lymphoma, leg type – Intravascular large B-cell lymphoma	**Fibrohistiocytic tumors** – DFSP and variants – Fibrosarcomatous DFSP – Myxoinflammatory fibroblastic sarcoma **Adipocytic tumors** – Atypical lipomatous tumor – Dedifferentiated liposarcoma – Pleomorphic liposarcoma **Smooth muscle tumors** – Atypical smooth muscle tumor/cutaneous leiomyosarcoma **Vascular tumors** – Cutaneous angiosarcoma – Hemangioendotheliomas – Kaposi sarcoma **Neural tumors** – Malignant peripheral nerve sheath tumor **Myo-pericytic tumors** – Malignant glomus tumor **Uncertain differentiation** – Atypical fibroxanthoma/pleomorphic dermal sarcoma – Myxofibrosarcoma – Epithelioid sarcoma

BCC Basal cell carcinoma, *SCC* Squamous cell carcinoma, *NOS* Not otherwise specified, *CSD* Cumulative sun-damage, *MF* Mycosis fungoides, *LPD* Lymphoproliferative disorder, *DFSP* Dermatofibrosarcoma protuberans
Adapted from Elder DE, Massi D, Scolyer RA, Willemze R, editors. WHO classification of skin tumours. Fourth ed. Lyon: IARC; 2018. p. 10–13

Basal Cell Carcinoma

Primary cutaneous BCC is a malignant cutaneous tumor characterized by the presence of lobules, columns, bands, or cords of basaloid cells. It is considered a tumor of follicular germ and arises from basal cells of the epidermis or hair follicle. It is the most prevalent malignant neoplasm accounting for about 75% of all NMSCs, with rates highest in Australia. UV radiation exposure, primarily UV-B spectrum (290–320 nm), is the most critical risk factor with tumors occurring commonly on sun-damaged skin of fair-skinned population (Fitzpatrick skin types I and II). The overall rate of BCC increases with the patient's age. In nevoid BCC syndrome (Gorlin syndrome), patients show germline mutations in the hedgehog signaling pathway (commonly patched gene PTCH1), and the onset of multiple BCCs can occur in younger patients. BCC can also develop within sites previously treated with radiation therapy (e.g., "field fire" BCC).

Histological Types

BCC is divided into various types or variants. These types are stratified according to low-risk (nonaggressive, indolent) and high-risk (aggressive) of recurrence. Superficial, nodular, pigmented, infundibulocystic, and fibroepithelial BCCs are grouped in the lower risk of recurrence category. Sclerosing/morpheaform, infiltrating, and micronodular BCCs; BCC with sarcomatoid differentiation; and basosquamous carcinoma are grouped in the high-risk of recurrence category.

Low-Risk of Recurrence BCC

The clinical appearance of BCC varies according to its type. Nodular BCC, the most common type, presents as an elevated pearly nodule or plaque associated with telangiectasia. It occurs more frequently on the head and neck, can be ulcerated or show cystic change, and is also known as a "rodent ulcer." Histopathologically, they show nodular dermal growth of large lobules of basaloid cells displaying peripheral palisading (Fig. 1.1a) and retraction artifact.

Superficial BCC generally presents as scaly, annular, erythematous patch or plaque, frequently occurring on the trunk. On microscopic analysis, they display superficial lobules of basaloid cells, which hang from the epidermis into the papillary dermis, surrounded by loose myxoid stroma.

Fibroepithelial BCC (of Pinkus) mostly occurs on the trunk and microscopically shows anastomosing basaloid strands surrounded by abundant stroma (Fig. 1.1b).

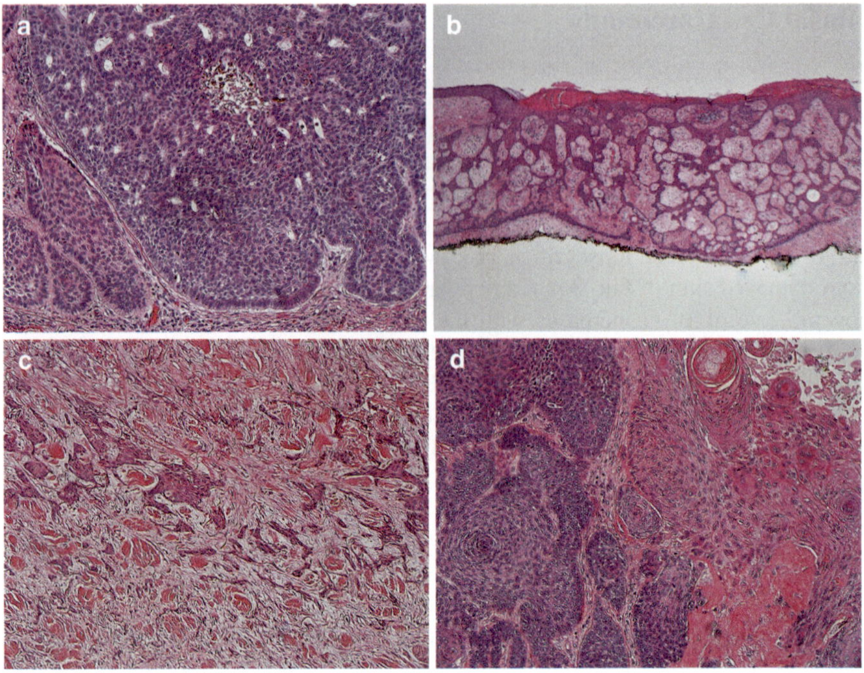

Fig. 1.1 (**a**) Nodular BCC formed by basaloid epithelial cells showing peripheral palisading (hematoxylin and eosin, ×100). (**b**) Fibroepithelial BCC formed by anastomosing interconnecting strands of basaloid cells (hematoxylin and eosin, ×25). (**c**) Sclerosing/morpheaform BCC formed by thin and jagged islands of basaloid cells infiltrating dense sclerotic collagenous stroma (hematoxylin and eosin, ×50). (**d**) Basosquamous carcinoma displaying features of both BCC and SCC (hematoxylin and eosin, ×100)

High-Risk of Recurrence BCC

In the high-risk of recurrence group, sclerosing/morpheaform and infiltrating types present as indurated, poorly defined plaque, displaying a scar-like appearance, often located on the upper trunk or head and neck. Microscopically, they are formed by thin and jagged strands, cords, and columns of basaloid cells that infiltrate the dermal collagen and may show perineural invasion (PI) with deep extension. Sclerosing/morpheaform type typically shows dense sclerotic collagenous or keloidal stroma (Fig. 1.1c). The histopathological differential diagnosis includes desmoplastic trichoepithelioma, the infiltrative pattern of SCC, and microcystic adnexal carcinoma.

Micronodular BCC is formed by micronodules about the size of follicular bulbs that show infiltration at the edges, permeate deep tissue, and may show PI.

Basosquamous carcinoma shows features of both BCC and SCC (Fig. 1.1d) [3]. It can display deep infiltrative growth pattern, transition zones with changes intermediate between the two entities, PI, and sometimes lymphovascular invasion (LVI). Tumors with a mixture of types, so-called composite BCC, are not uncommon. The identified highest risk component best determines the risk status in the composite type.

Immunohistochemical Profile

The diagnosis and typing of BCC are usually made on microscopic analysis, and additional ancillary studies are only required in complicated cases. BCCs are positive for Bcl-2 and BerEp4 stains. They are negative for S100, EMA, and CEA and show fewer CK20-positive cells. BerEp4 and EMA can be seen in BCC and SCC components in basosquamous carcinoma, respectively.

Predictive Parameters and Prognosis

Histopathological reports, including data items such as type, maximum tumor dimension, depth of invasion (DOI) and deep invasion (including involvement of cartilage or bone), and PI, are helpful for risk assessment and management (Table 1.2) [4]. The American Joint Committee on Cancer (AJCC) Eighth Edition Manual has no separate designated staging system for BCC, and it is incorporated with other NMSCs.

BCC is a locally invasive tumor with increased morbidity in deeply invasive and large neglected tumors. The high-risk of recurrence is chiefly attributed to the type of BCC and tends to be more common on sites where it is difficult to achieve adequate margins (e.g., nose or nasolabial fold). PI correlates with a higher risk of local recurrence. Post-radiotherapy local recurrences are usually more aggressive and infiltrative.

Metastatic risk is minimal in BCC (estimated between 0.0028% and 0.5%) [5] and is generally seen in large, neglected, recurrent tumors or basosquamous morphology. The metastatic rate of basosquamous carcinoma (5–9%) is similar to SCC, occurring in regional lymph nodes followed by lungs. Although basosquamous carcinoma is considered a type of BCC, its behavior suggests that it has more similarities to cutaneous SCC.

The main emphasis of treatment is on the excision of tumor with margin control (via conventional surgical excisions or Mohs micrographic surgery). Mohs micrographic surgery provides excellent cure rates for high-risk and recurrent BCCs and BCCs involving cosmetically sensitive sites. For conventional skin excisions, peripheral and deep margin reporting as involved, uninvolved, and uninvolved but close (for less than 1 mm) helps manage the clearance of tumors.

Table 1.2 Basal cell carcinoma: Synopsis

Low-risk of recurrence types
Superficial BCC
Nodular BCC
Pigmented BCC
Infundibulocystic BCC
Fibroepithelial BCC
High-risk of recurrence types
Sclerosing/morpheaform BCC
Infiltrating BCC
Micronodular BCC
Basosquamous carcinoma
BCC with sarcomatoid differentiation
Clinical presentation
Most common malignant neoplasm, about 75% of all NMSCs
UV radiation exposure, sun-damaged skin of fair-skinned, sites with prior radiation therapy
Nodular type: elevated pearly nodule with telangiectasia, head and neck
Superficial type: erythematous patch or plaque, trunk
Sclerosing/morpheaform and infiltrating types: indurated, poorly defined plaque, scar-like appearance, upper trunk or head and neck
Associated heritable syndromes
Nevoid BCC syndrome
Bazex syndrome
Rombo syndrome
Multiple hereditary infundibulocystic BCC
Xeroderma pigmentosum
Histopathology and immunohistochemical profile
Lobules of basaloid cells, peripheral palisading, retraction artifact
Sclerosing/morpheaform type: thin infiltrating cords and columns, sclerotic collagenous stroma
Micronodular type: micronodules size of follicular bulbs, infiltrating edges
Basosquamous carcinoma: features of both BCC and SCC
Positive for Bcl-2 and BerEp4 stains
Predictive parameters
Risk determinants:
– Type, site (nose, eyelids/around eyes, ears), poorly defined borders, recurrent tumors, immunosuppression, prior radiotherapy, maximum tumor dimension (more than 2.0 cm), DOI (more than 6 mm), deep invasion beyond subcutis, PI
Locally invasive tumor
Metastasis rarely occurs, more frequent in basosquamous carcinoma

NMSC Non-melanoma skin cancer, *BCC* Basal cell carcinoma, *UV* Ultraviolet, *SCC* Squamous cell carcinoma, *DOI* Depth of invasion, *PI* Perineural invasion

Cutaneous Squamous Cell Carcinoma

Primary cutaneous SCC is the second most common form of cutaneous malignancy, with about 2500 deaths annually in the USA. It arises from epidermal keratinocytes and is most frequent on the chronically sun-exposed skin of the fair-skinned. The head and neck area is the most common site, the incidence is higher in men, and the affected individuals are usually over the age of 40 years.

Risk Factors

Major risk factors include UV radiation exposure, immunosuppressive states (solid-organ transplant recipients, human immunodeficiency virus), infections (human papillomavirus, epidermodysplasia verruciformis), chemical carcinogens (e.g., arsenic, coal tar), chronic inflammation and wounds (e.g., sinus tracts, burn scars), cutaneous inflammatory conditions (e.g., lichen planus, vitiligo), adverse treatment effect (e.g., immunotherapy, radiation therapy), and genetic disorders (e.g., xeroderma pigmentosum, oculocutaneous albinism, dystrophic epidermolysis bullosa, multiple familial keratoacanthomas of Ferguson-Smith type).

Clinical Presentation

SCC clinically presents as a hyperkeratotic patch or plaque, papule, or nodule, which may ulcerate with progression. SCC with PI can be accompanied by abnormal sensations or pain. Larger cranial nerves can be involved, especially the facial nerve and the second division of the trigeminal nerve. The keratoacanthoma type displays a cup-shaped appearance with a central keratin plug and has proliferative, mature, and regressing stages of evolution. Verrucous SCC, clinically displaying cauliflower-like growth, can occur both in the oral cavity and primarily skin of the anogenital region (giant condyloma of Buschke-Löwenstein) and palms or soles (epithelioma cuniculatum). Marjolin's ulcer is a term for SCCs developing in burn scars and long-standing lower extremity wounds.

Histopathology and Histological Types

Microscopically, SCC typically shows origin and attachment to the surface epidermis with frequent presence of precursor lesions (e.g., actinic keratosis, Bowen's disease). Keratinocyte atypia is present and varies from minimal to marked, depending on the type of SCC and degree of differentiation (Fig. 1.2a, b). Keratinization, infiltrative growth with desmoplastic stromal reaction, and PI are noted. SCC has multiple histological types: conventional, acantholytic, keratoacanthoma, spindle cell, verrucous, pseudovascular, adenosquamous, clear cell, and lymphoepithelioma-like. Keratoacanthoma type shows the crateriform architecture, intraepithelial microabscesses, and features of regression. Verrucous SCC characteristically displays an endophytic growth pattern with pushing borders and minimal cytological atypia.

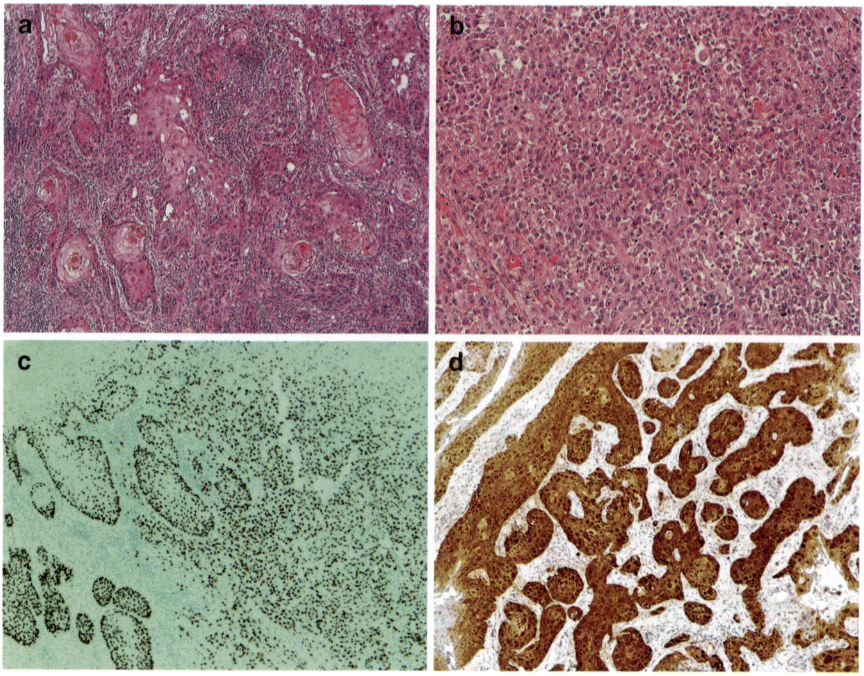

Fig. 1.2 (**a**) Infiltrative growth of keratinizing jagged nests of cutaneous SCC (hematoxylin and eosin, ×100). (**b**) Sheets of poorly differentiated areas in cutaneous SCC (hematoxylin and eosin, ×200). (**c**) Nuclear positivity with p40 marker in cutaneous SCC (p40, ×40). (**d**) p16 block positivity noted in SCC of the nail unit (p16, ×100)

Immunohistochemical Profile

Immunohistochemistry is usually unnecessary and is used only in complicated cases such as spindle cell type and poorly or undifferentiated lesions. SCCs are positive for AE1/AE3, 34BE12, EMA, p40 (Fig. 1.2c), p63, and CK5/6 markers. They are typically negative for S100 and BerEp4 stains. AE1/AE3 can be negative in spindle cell type, and p40 or p63 stains are usually required for diagnosis. p16 stain can be employed as a surrogate marker to assess high-risk human papillomavirus infection (Fig. 1.2d).

Predictive Parameters and Prognosis

Unfavorable prognostic clinical parameters include immunosuppressive states and high-risk anatomic sites (i.e., ear, cutaneous lip). Cutaneous lip SCC has a metastatic rate of 10–14%, and ear SCC has a rate of 11%. Unfavorable pathological predictive factors include tumor size (more than 2 cm), DOI (more than 2 mm), Clark level (more than IV), poorly differentiated or undifferentiated, spindle cell or adenosquamous morphology, and PI or LVI [6]. PI is associated with higher local recurrence rate, lymph node, and distant metastasis.

Superficial SCCs are usually indolent; however, SCCs do tend to have a greater tendency to recur and metastasize than BCCs. The overall rate of metastasis is 2.3–5.2%. Most keratoacanthoma type SCCs resolve by regression; however, subungual and central facial lesions can show local aggressive behavior and destruction of underlying structures. Verrucous SCC is locally aggressive with a high local recurrence rate; however, metastasis usually does not occur unless the lesion dedifferentiates to a more aggressive form. Such aggressive transformation in the verrucous type has been reported after treating tumors with radiation therapy. Marjolin's ulcers behave aggressively, with a high rate of metastasis, with 54% of metastatic lesions occurring on lower extremities and the overall metastatic rate between 20% and 30% [7].

Pathological Staging

AJCC (Eighth Edition) staging of cutaneous SCC of head and neck is based on maximum tumor size (cutoff 2 cm and 4 cm), deep invasion beyond the subcutaneous fat, PI (nerve lying deeper than dermis or nerve measuring 0.1 mm or larger in caliber), cortical bone or skull base invasion, degree and size of lymph node metastasis, and systemic metastasis (Table 1.3) [8]. Brigham and Women's Hospital classification system for cutaneous SCC provides a substitute staging system [9]. Excision of tumors with margin control (via conventional surgical excisions or Mohs micrographic surgery) is performed for resectable tumors. Peripheral and deep margin reporting with distance to closest margins is recommended for skin excisions.

Table 1.3 Cutaneous squamous cell carcinoma: Synopsis and AJCC Pathological Staging (Eighth Edition) of cSCC-HN

Synopsis
Clinical presentation
Chronically sun-exposed skin, fair-skinned, head and neck
Hyperkeratotic lesion, may arise with precursor lesions (e.g., actinic keratosis, Bowen's disease)
PI: paresthesia or pain
Keratoacanthoma type: cup-shaped appearance, central keratin plug
Verrucous type: oral cavity, anogenital, palms/soles, cauliflower-like
Marjolin's ulcer: SCC in chronic wounds and ulcers
Histological types
Conventional, acantholytic, keratoacanthoma, spindle cell, verrucous, pseudovascular, adenosquamous, clear cell, and lymphoepithelioma-like
Immunohistochemical profile
AE1/AE3+, 34BE12+, EMA+, p40+, p63+, CK5/6+
S100−, BerEp4−
p16: surrogate marker for high-risk HPV
Unfavorable clinical predictive parameters
Immunosuppressive states and high-risk anatomic sites (i.e., ear, cutaneous lip)
Unfavorable pathological predictive parameters
Tumor size, DOI, poor differentiation, PI, and LVI
Staging
AJCC of cSCC-HN
Brigham and Women's Hospital classification system
Primary tumor
pTX: cannot be determined
pTis: in situ
pT1: tumor smaller than or equal to 2 cm
pT2: tumor larger than 2 cm, but smaller than or equal to 4 cm
pT3: tumor larger than 4 cm or PI or deep invasion or minor bone erosion
pT4a: tumor with gross cortical bone/marrow invasion
pT4b: tumor with skull base invasion and/or skull base foramen involvement
Regional LN metastasis
pNX: cannot be determined
pN0: no regional LN metastasis
pN1: metastasis in single IPL LN, 3 cm or smaller, and negative ENE
pN2a: metastasis in single IPL LN, 3 cm or smaller and positive ENE; or single IPL LN, larger than 3 cm but not larger than 6 cm and negative ENE
pN2b: metastases in multiple IPL LN(s), none larger than 6 cm and negative ENE
pN2c: metastases in BL or CNL LN(s), none larger than 6 cm and negative ENE
pN3a: metastasis in a LN larger than 6 cm and negative ENE
pN3b: metastasis in single IPL LN larger than 3 cm and positive ENE; or multiple IPL, CNL, or BL LNs any with positive ENE; or single CNL LN of any size and positive ENE
Distant metastasis
pM0: no distant metastasis
pM1: distant metastasis

AJCC American Joint Committee on Cancer, *cSCC-HN* Cutaneous squamous cell carcinoma of the head and neck, *PI* Perineural invasion, *SCC* Squamous cell carcinoma, *HPV* Human papillomavirus, *DOI* Depth of invasion, *LVI* Lymphovascular invasion, *LN* Lymph node, *IPL* Ipsilateral, *ENE* Extranodal extension, *BL* Bilateral, *CNL* Contralateral

Pathological Staging: Adapted from Califano JA, Lydiatt WM, Nehal KS, O'Sullivan B, Schmults C, Seethala RR, et al. Cutaneous squamous cell carcinoma of the head and neck. In: Amin MB, Edge SB, Greene FL, et al., editors. AJCC Cancer Staging Manual. Eighth ed. New York: Springer; 2017. p. 171–181

Merkel Cell Carcinoma

Merkel cell carcinoma (MCC), also known as primary cutaneous neuroendocrine or trabecular carcinoma, mainly affects the sun-damaged skin of elderly fair-skinned patients. It is an uncommon but often lethal and aggressive malignancy. The median age at diagnosis is about 75 years, more common in men, and there is an association with immunosuppressive states. The incidence is higher in patients with chronic lymphocytic leukemia, HIV infection, and organ transplant. The incidence of MCC has tripled in the past 20 years, primarily due to improved diagnosis, increased numbers of immunosuppressed patients, and an increase in the number of older individuals.

Clinical Presentation

The neoplasm favors the head and neck and presents as a rapidly expanding firm skin-colored nodule. AEIOU acronym, representing Asymptomatic, Expanding rapidly, Immune suppressed, Older than 50 years, and UV-exposed fair skin, is used to help remember salient clinical parameters. The primary tumor can regress, and nodal or visceral metastasis can develop without detectable primary MCC.

Histogenesis and Types

In 1972, Toker first described five cases of trabecular carcinoma of the skin. In 1980, DeWolff-Peeters et al. named it Merkel cell carcinoma based on features shared between this neoplasm and normal Merkel cells (mechanoreceptors) in the skin. In the 1980s, the diagnosis of MCC was rarely made. However, reported incidence increased significantly in the 1990s with broader immunohistochemical stain (such as CK20) utilization. The cell of origin of this tumor is indefinite. The presumptive cell of origin includes cutaneous Merkel cells, epithelial progenitors, fibroblast and dermal stem cells, and pre-B/pro-B cells [10]. Recently, two types or subsets of MCC have been described. The first is due to clonal integration of Merkel cell polyomavirus (MCPyV). It is the more common subset accounting for about 80% of tumors. The second less common one is related to UV radiation exposure-induced damage.

Histopathology

MCC usually presents as a cutaneous dermal based round blue cell tumor (Fig. 1.3a). The architecture can be nodular and infiltrating, arranged mainly in sheets and nests. The tumor is formed by small to intermediate, round to oval cells of uniform size with vesicular nucleus displaying fine granular salt and pepper chromatin. Mitoses and apoptotic bodies are numerous, and LVI is frequent (Fig. 1.3b). The histopathological differential diagnosis includes metastatic neuroendocrine carcinoma of the extracutaneous site (e.g., lung), BCC, lymphoma, or sarcomas with round blue cell morphology (e.g., Ewing sarcoma). Spontaneous regression of primary tumor and satellite metastasis in surrounding skin can occur. Collision tumors (e.g., with SCC) and biphenotypic combined MCC do occur (Fig. 1.3c). MCPyV is generally absent in combined tumors.

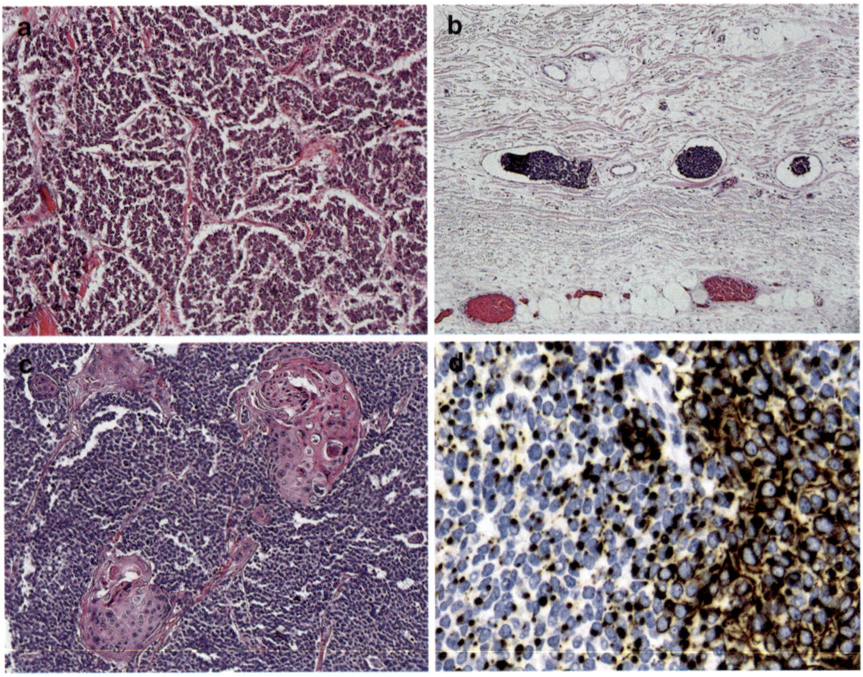

Fig. 1.3 (**a**) Sheets and nests of dermal based round blue cells in MCC (hematoxylin and eosin, ×100). (**b**) Lymphovascular invasion displayed by MCC (hematoxylin and eosin, ×40). (**c**) Biphenotypic mixed neuroendocrine and squamous differentiation in combined MCC (hematoxylin and eosin, ×200). (**d**) Perinuclear dot-like pattern of positivity with CK20 in MCC (CK20, ×400)

Immunohistochemical Profile

MCC is positive for neuroendocrine immunohistochemical stains (e.g., synaptophysin, chromogranin A, and CD56) and epithelial markers (e.g., AE1/AE3, CAM5.2, EMA, Ber-Ep4, and CK20). CK20 positivity is seen in more than 90% of tumors displaying characteristic perinuclear dot-like pattern (Fig. 1.3d) highlighting aggregates of intermediate keratin filaments. CK7, TTF-1, LCA, and S100 stains are typically negative. CM2B4 antibody can be used to confirm the presence of MCPyV large T-antigen. Also, as immunostains increase the sensitivity of identifying occult lymph node metastasis, they are recommended for lymph node evaluation.

Predictive Parameters and Pathological Staging

Maximum clinical tumor diameter and extent of local invasion, tumor thickness, mitotic rate, tumor-infiltrating lymphocytes, nodular or infiltrative growth pattern, pure or combined type, LVI, and microscopic satellitosis or in-transit metastasis are data elements which are included in the pathology report. For skin excisions, distance of the tumor from closest peripheral and deep specimen margins is reported. AJCC (Eighth Edition) staging is based on maximum clinical tumor diameter and extracutaneous invasion, degree of regional lymph node or in-transit metastasis, and systemic metastasis (Table 1.4) [11]. MCPyV-negative tumors tend to have a worse prognosis than MCPyV-positive tumors. The 5-year overall survival rate of MCC is about 51% (localized disease), 35% (regional metastasis), and 14% (distant metastasis).

Table 1.4 Merkel cell carcinoma: Synopsis and AJCC Pathological Staging (Eighth Edition)

Synopsis
Clinical presentation
AEIOU: Asymptomatic, Expanding rapidly, Immune suppressed, Older than 50 years, UV-exposed fair skin
Pathogenesis
Clonal integration of MCPyV, UV-induced
Histopathology
Round blue cell tumor, salt-and-pepper chromatin, pure and combined types
Immunohistochemical profile
Neuroendocrine markers (synaptophysin+, chromogranin A+, CD56+)
Epithelial markers (AE1/AE3+, CAM5.2+, EMA+, Ber-Ep4+, CK20+), perinuclear dot-like pattern
CM2B4 (confirm presence of MCPyV large T-antigen)
Prognosis
5-Year overall survival rate: 51% (localized disease), 35% (regional metastasis), and 14% (distant metastasis)
MCPyV-negative tumors: worse prognosis

(continued)

Table 1.4 (continued)

Synopsis
Primary tumor
pTX: cannot be determined pT0: no evidence of primary tumor pTis: in situ pT1: maximum CTD less than or equal to 2 cm pT2: maximum CTD greater than 2 but less than or equal to 5 cm pT3: maximum CTD greater than 5 cm pT4: tumor invades fascia, muscle, cartilage, or bone
Regional LN metastasis
pNX: cannot be determined pN0: no regional LN metastasis pN1: metastasis in regional LN(s) – pN1a (sentinel LN): clinically occult LN metastasis, sentinel LN examination only – pN1a: clinically occult LN metastasis, lymph node dissection performed – pN1b: clinically/radiologically detected LN metastasis, confirmed by microscopic examination pN2: in-transit metastasis, without LN metastasis pN3: in-transit metastasis, with LN metastasis
Distant metastasis
pM0: no distant metastasis pM1: distant metastasis – pM1a: distant skin, distant subcutaneous tissue, or distant LN(s) metastasis – pM1b: lung metastasis – pM1c: all other site(s) metastasis

AJCC American Joint Committee on Cancer, *MCPyV* Merkel cell polyomavirus, *UV* Ultraviolet, *CTD* Clinical tumor diameter, *LN* Lymph node

Pathological Staging: Adapted from Bichakjian CK, Nghiem P, Johnson T, Wright WL, Sober AJ. Merkel cell carcinoma. In: Amin MB, Edge SB, Greene FL, et al., editors. AJCC Cancer Staging Manual. Eighth ed. New York: Springer; 2017. p. 549–62

Cutaneous Melanoma

The incidence of melanoma has been increasing rapidly worldwide. It originates from melanocytes and, apart from the skin, can arise in other parts of the body, such as intraoral, sinonasal, anogenital, uveal, and conjunctival.

Histological Types

Cutaneous melanoma has many types (Table 1.1). The major ones are superficial spreading melanoma, lentigo maligna melanoma, nodular melanoma, acral melanoma, and desmoplastic melanoma. The 2018 WHO classification has presented a more refined classification built on epidemiological, clinical, pathological, and genomic findings [12]. Due to the presence of multiple types, melanoma can have diverse clinical presentations. The ABCDE acronym characterizes the flat lesions:

Asymmetry, Border irregularity, Color variegation, Diameter more than 6 mm, and Evolving. The microscopic features include asymmetry and poor circumscription, absence of maturation, intraepidermal pagetoid scatter, nuclear pleomorphism, and intraepidermal and dermal mitosis.

Superficial Spreading Melanoma

Superficial spreading melanoma (low cumulative sun-damage (CSD) melanoma) represents the most common type in fair-skinned, occurring commonly on the back and legs in males and females, respectively. It presents with an irregular pigmented macular lesion (radial growth phase, RGP), which subsequently develops a papule or nodule (vertical growth phase, VGP). Microscopically, in situ and invasive components are formed by epithelioid melanocytes showing marked intraepidermal pagetoid "buck-shot" scatter (Fig. 1.4a). In about one-third of cases, an associated benign nevus is identified. Chromosomal abnormalities are frequent, and common genetic mutations include BRAF p.V600E, CDKN2A, and TERT promoter.

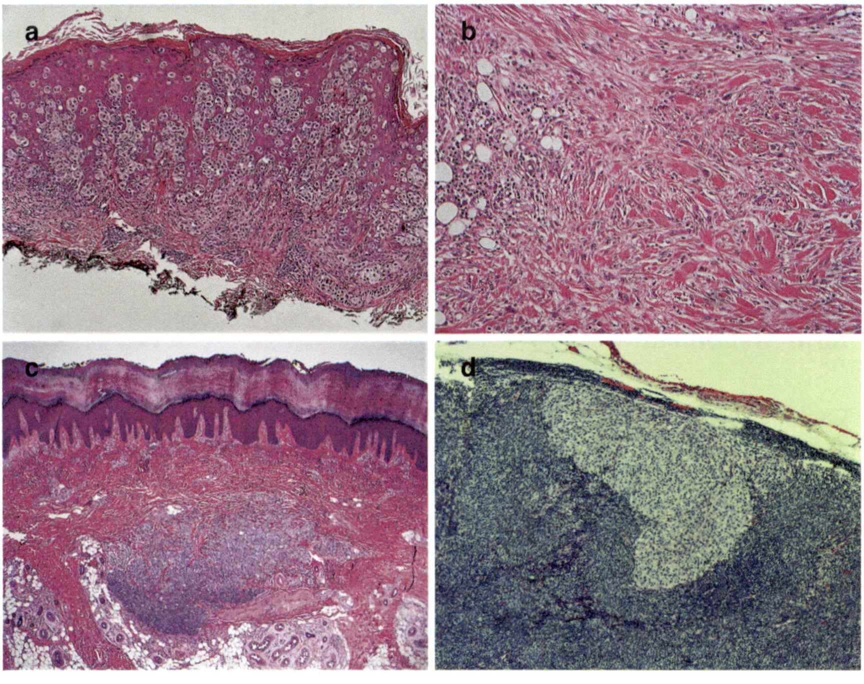

Fig. 1.4 (**a**) In situ component of superficial spreading melanoma formed by epithelioid melanocytes showing marked intraepidermal pagetoid "buck-shot" scatter (hematoxylin and eosin, ×100). (**b**) Pure desmoplastic melanoma formed by spindled melanoma cells embedded in a dense fibrous scar-like stroma (hematoxylin and eosin, ×200). (**c**) In-transit metastasis in association with an acral melanoma (hematoxylin and eosin, ×25). (**d**) Subcapsular metastasis of melanoma in a sentinel LN (hematoxylin and eosin, ×50)

Lentigo Maligna Melanoma

Lentigo maligna melanoma (high-CSD melanoma) typically arises on the chronically sun-damaged skin of the elderly, occurring in an older population as compared to low-CSD melanomas. It presents as a slowly evolving irregularly pigmented patch or plaque (RGP), most frequently on the skin of the head and neck. An invasive tumor (VGP) often occurs after a long interval, with a latency period ranging from months to decades. Microscopically, the in situ component is characterized by intraepidermal contiguous lentiginous and nested atypical melanocytes with dermal solar elastosis. The peripheral borders are indistinct; appendageal involvement is commonly seen, and pagetoid scatter is less prominent. Genomically, they have a very high mutation burden, with mutations carrying a UV radiation signature. They show loss of NF1 and mutations of NRAS, non-pV600E BRAF, KIT, and TERT promotor.

Nodular Melanoma

Nodular melanoma represents VGP melanoma arising in the absence of a developed RGP. It presents as a nodular tumor, often ulcerated, with no adjacent RGP. Most nodular melanomas are thick tumors on presentation, so they are associated with poor prognosis. Microscopically, they are defined by no evidence of an in situ component beyond three adjacent rete ridges and form a tumorigenic component in the dermis. Genomically, they represent a heterogeneous group whose profile overlaps with other melanoma types. It likely represents an accelerated growth pattern of other types rather than a distinct genomic group.

Acral Melanoma

Acral melanoma occurs on non-hair-bearing acral skin, most commonly affecting the heel. Subungual variants are also encountered, about 20% of acral type, usually involving the great toe and thumb. This type is less common in fair-skinned, accounting for less than 10% of all melanomas. The acral type is the most frequent form of melanoma in colored races. Microscopically, the RGP component is lentiginous and can be subtle. The VGP component can be spindled, epithelioid, or desmoplastic and may display heterologous (metaplastic) differentiation. Genomically, they lack UV radiation signature and show KIT, BRAF, and NRAS mutations.

Desmoplastic Melanoma

Desmoplastic melanoma usually presents as an infiltrative scar-like plaque or nodular amelanotic lesion on chronically sun-damaged skin of the head and neck in the elderly. Local recurrence is more common than non-desmoplastic melanomas, although the pure form metastasizes less frequently. Microscopically, it is formed by spindled melanoma cells embedded in a dense fibrous stroma (Fig. 1.4b). It can have a surface lentigo maligna-like in situ component; however, about half the lesions lack a discernable intraepidermal component. It often shows neurotropism (about 30% of cases). Neurotropism is best assessed at the lesion's periphery, and entrapment of nerves in the primary tumor mass does not constitute neurotropism. The lesional cells can be negative for HMB45 and Mart-1 stains; however, S100 and SOX10 are positive. It has pure and mixed (with non-desmoplastic melanoma) histological subtypes [13], with pure form displaying a low incidence of regional lymph node metastasis and a more favorable prognosis. When metastasis occurs, the lung is the more common initial location. Genomically, they have UV radiation signature with a very high mutation burden. They frequently harbor NF1 mutations.

Immunohistochemical Profile

A wide variety of immunohistochemical stains are used to characterize melanocytic proliferations. These include differentiation markers (e.g., S100, HMB45, Melan-A/MART1, SOX10, MITF, tyrosinase), biomarkers (e.g., Ki-67 (MIB-1), PHH3, p16, PRAME, BAP1, ALK, NTRK), mutation antigens (e.g., BRAF-V600E, RASQ61R (NRASQ61R), HRAS), and those used to assess immune response score (e.g., PD1, PD-L1). A panel of immunohistochemical stains (e.g., S100, HMB45, MART1) is usually performed on sentinel lymph nodes to improve the detection of metastasis [14].

Predictive Parameters and Pathological Staging

Histopathologic parameters like tumor thickness (Breslow thickness), ulceration, histological type, Clark level, mitotic rate, satellitosis and in-transit metastasis (Fig. 1.4c), LVI, neurotropism, regression, and tumor-infiltrating lymphocytes are required elements in pathology reports of melanoma. Tumor thickness is the main prognostic factor for localized primary melanoma. It is measured with the granular layer of epidermis or base of the ulcer as the upper reference point and the deepest point of the invasive tumor as the lower reference point. Margin assessment with the distance of melanoma from the closest peripheral and deep margins is reported. AJCC staging is based on tumor thickness and ulceration, degree of regional lymph node (Fig. 1.4d) or in-transit metastasis, and systemic metastasis (Table 1.5) [15].

Table 1.5 Cutaneous melanoma: Synopsis and AJCC Pathological Staging (Eighth Edition)

Synopsis
Clinical presentation ABCDE: Asymmetry, Border irregularity, Color variegation, Diameter more than 6 mm, Evolving **Histological types** Superficial spreading melanoma, lentigo maligna melanoma, desmoplastic melanoma, acral melanoma, nodular melanoma, nevoid melanoma, melanoma arising in a blue nevus, melanoma arising in a giant congenital nevus, Spitz melanoma **Immunohistochemical profile** Differentiation markers (S100, HMB45, Melan-A/MART1, SOX10, MITF) Biomarkers (Ki-67, PHH3, p16, PRAME, BAP1, ALK, NTRK) Mutation antigens (BRAF-V600E, RASQ61R, HRAS) **Predictive parameters** Tumor thickness, ulceration, type, Clark level, mitotic rate, IT-S-M, lymphovascular invasion, neurotropism, regression, tumor-infiltrating lymphocytes
Primary tumor
pTX: cannot be determined pT0: no evidence of primary tumor pT1a: melanoma less than 0.8 mm in thickness, no ulceration pT1b: melanoma less than 0.8 mm with ulceration or melanoma 0.8–1.0 mm with/without ulceration pT2a: melanoma greater than 1.0–2.0 mm, no ulceration pT2b: melanoma greater than 1.0–2.0 mm, with ulceration pT3a: melanoma greater than 2.0–4.0 mm, no ulceration pT3b: melanoma greater than 2.0–4.0 mm, with ulceration pT4a: melanoma greater than 4.0 mm, no ulceration pT4b: melanoma greater than 4.0 mm, with ulceration
Regional LN metastasis
pNX: cannot be determined pN0: no regional LN metastasis pN1a: one CO tumor-involved LN, with no IT-S-M pN1b: one CD tumor-involved LN, with no IT-S-M pN1c: presence of IT-S-M, with no regional LN involvement pN2a: 2–3 CO tumor-involved LNs, with no IT-S-M pN2b: 2–3 tumor-involved LNs, at least one CD, with no IT-S-M pN2c: 1 CO or CD tumor-involved LN, with IT-S-M pN3a: 4 or more CO tumor-involved LNs, with no IT-S-M pN3b: 4 or more tumor-involved LNs, at least one CD, with no IT-S-M pN3c: 2 or more CO or CD tumor-involved LNs, with IT-S-M or any number of matted LNs with IT-S-M
Distant metastasis
pM0: no distant metastasis pM1: distant metastasis – pM1a: distant metastasis in skin, subcutaneous tissue, soft tissue, non-regional LN – pM1b: distant metastasis to lung, with or without M1a site – pM1c: distant metastasis to non-CNS visceral site, with or without M1a or M1b site – pM1d: distant metastasis to CNS, with or without M1a, M1b or M1c site

AJCC American Joint Committee on Cancer, *LN* Lymph node, *IT-S-M* In-transit/satellite/microsatellite, *CO* Clinically occult, *CD* Clinically detected, *CNS* Central nervous system

Pathological Staging: Adapted from Gershenwald JE, Scolyer RA, Hess KR, Thompson JF, Long GV, Ross MI, et al. Melanoma of the skin. In: Amin MB, Edge SB, Greene FL, et al. editors. AJCC Cancer Staging Manual. Eighth ed. New York: Springer; 2017. p. 563–85

Other Cutaneous Malignancies

Other main categories of skin malignancies include malignant appendageal tumors, primary cutaneous lymphomas, and malignant cutaneous soft tissue tumors. Each category contains a broad spectrum of neoplasms with detailed classifications (Table 1.1) [1, 2].

Malignant Appendageal Tumor

Malignant appendageal or adnexal tumors are uncommon and are further subdivided into four groups: tumors with eccrine and apocrine, follicle, and sebaceous differentiation and site-specific tumors.

Microcystic adnexal carcinoma, usually located on the face (especially the upper lip), is deeply infiltrative dermal tumor with PI commonly present. They are locally aggressive tumors with a propensity for recurrence.

Pilomatrical carcinoma shows matrical differentiation and mainly occurs on the face of middle-aged to older men. It shows both nuclear and cytoplasmic staining for the beta-catenin marker. They show high local recurrence rates and are associated with regional lymph nodes and visceral metastasis.

Sebaceous carcinoma occurs on periocular and extraocular sites, with about 50% occurring on the eyelid. They can be clinically confused with chalazion, which results in diagnostic delay. They clinically behave aggressively with a 20–25% risk of distant metastasis.

Mammary Paget's disease represents a retrograde extension of breast carcinoma into the epidermis. In more than 95% of cases, underlying breast carcinoma is present. Extramammary Paget's disease can be primary (originating in the skin) or secondary (intraepidermal spread of underlying carcinoma). The majority of cases are primary, and it typically occurs in anogenital sites (especially the vulva). Microscopically, they show the presence of intraepidermal tumor cells displaying prominent pagetoid scatter.

Primary Cutaneous Lymphoma

Primary cutaneous lymphomas are subdivided into cutaneous T-cell lymphomas (CTCLs) and cutaneous B-cell lymphomas [2]. They represent a heterogeneous group with 75–80% in the T-cell category.

Mycosis fungoides is the most common type of primary cutaneous lymphoma, constituting about 50% of all primary skin lymphomas and about 60% of all primary CTCLs. Folliculotropic, pagetoid reticulosis, and granulomatous slack skin types are considered variants of mycosis fungoides.

The second most common group is primary cutaneous CD30-positive lymphoproliferative disorders, comprising about 25% of all primary CTCLs. They include multiple histological subtypes of lymphomatoid papulosis and primary cutaneous anaplastic large lymphoma.

Histopathologically, accurate categorization and distinction from benign dermatoses/pseudolymphomas require ancillary studies. Clinical correlation, histopathological analysis, a panel of immunohistochemical markers, and molecular genetic studies (e.g., gene rearrangement studies) are all utilized to arrive at the correct diagnosis.

Malignant Cutaneous Soft Tissue Tumor

Malignant cutaneous soft tissue tumors or cutaneous sarcomas are a diverse group further subdivided into fibrohistiocytic, adipocytic, vascular, neural, smooth muscle, myo-pericytic, and uncertain differentiation tumors. Due to their specific clinical behavior, malignant cutaneous soft tissue tumors must be discerned from their deep soft tissue counterparts.

Dermatofibrosarcoma protuberans is a fibrohistiocytic neoplasm usually occurring on the trunk. It is typically characterized by CD34-positive dermal spindle cell proliferation, showing a storiform pattern of growth and honeycomb permeation of subcutaneous fat. In about 10% of cases, fibrosarcomatous transformation occurs. These tumors have a high risk of local recurrence, and the fibrosarcomatous variant has metastatic potential.

Atypical fibroxanthoma usually arises on chronically sun-damaged skin in the elderly fair-skinned population. They are dermal tumors displaying high cellularity, striking cytological atypia, and atypical mitoses. Immunostains are typically utilized to exclude melanoma and high-grade squamous cell carcinoma. Larger lesion with similar morphology, which invades subcutaneous fat and deeper soft tissue and shows necrosis, and PI or LVI, should be classified as pleomorphic dermal sarcoma. If strict criteria are used, most atypical fibroxanthomas behave in a benign fashion. Pleomorphic dermal sarcoma shows more aggressive behavior with a higher risk of local recurrence and regional and distant metastasis.

References

1. Elder DE, Massi D, Scolyer RA, Willemze R, editors. WHO classification of skin tumours. 4th ed. Lyon: IARC; 2018. p. 10–3.
2. Willemze R, Cerroni L, Kempf W, Berti E, Facchetti F, Swerdlow SH, et al. The 2018 update of the WHO-EORTC classification for primary cutaneous lymphomas. Blood. 2019;133:1703–14. https://doi.org/10.1182/blood-2018-11-881268.
3. Wermker K, Roknic N, Goessling K, Klein M, Schulze HJ, Hallermann C. Basosquamous carcinoma of the head and neck: clinical and histologic characteristics and their impact on disease progression. Neoplasia. 2015;17:301–5. https://doi.org/10.1016/j.neo.2015.01.007.
4. Nasr I, McGrath EJ, Harwood CA, Botting J, Buckley P, Budny PG, et al. British Association of Dermatologists guidelines for the management of adults with basal cell carcinoma 2021. Br J Dermatol. 2021;185:899–920. https://doi.org/10.1111/bjd.20524.
5. Malone JP, Fedok FG, Belchis DA, Maloney ME. Basal cell carcinoma metastatic to the parotid: report of a new case and review of the literature. Ear Nose Throat J. 2000;79:511–5.
6. Newlands C, Currie R, Memon A, Whitaker S, Woolford T. Non-melanoma skin cancer: United Kingdom national multidisciplinary guidelines. J Laryngol Otol. 2016;130:S125–32. https://doi.org/10.1017/S0022215116000554.
7. Pekarek B, Buck S, Osher L. A comprehensive review on Marjolin's ulcers: diagnosis and treatment. J Am Col Certif Wound Spec. 2011;3:60–4. https://doi.org/10.1016/j.jcws.2012.04.001.
8. Califano JA, Lydiatt WM, Nehal KS, O'Sullivan B, Schmults C, Seethala RR, et al. Cutaneous squamous cell carcinoma of the head and neck. In: Amin MB, Edge SB, Greene FL, et al., editors. AJCC cancer staging manual. 8th ed. New York: Springer; 2017. p. 171–81.
9. Ruiz ES, Karia PS, Besaw R, Schmults CD. Performance of the American Joint Committee on Cancer Staging Manual, 8th Edition vs the Brigham and Women's Hospital Tumor Classification System for cutaneous squamous cell carcinoma. JAMA Dermatol. 2019;155:819–25. https://doi.org/10.1001/jamadermatol.2019.0032.
10. Kervarrec T, Samimi M, Guyétant S, Sarma B, Chéret J, Blanchard E, et al. Histogenesis of Merkel cell carcinoma: a comprehensive review. Front Oncol. 2019;9:451. https://doi.org/10.3389/fonc.2019.00451.
11. Bichakjian CK, Nghiem P, Johnson T, Wright WL, Sober AJ. Merkel cell carcinoma. In: Amin MB, Edge SB, Greene FL, et al., editors. AJCC Cancer Staging Manual. 8th ed. New York: Springer; 2017. p. 549–62.
12. Bastian BC, de la Fouchardiere A, Elder DE, Gerami P, Lazar AJ, Massi D, et al. Genomic landscape of melanoma. In: Elder DR, Massi D, Scolyer RA, Willemze R, editors. WHO classification of skin tumours. 4th ed. Lyon: IARC; 2018. p. 74–5.
13. Busam KJ, Mujumdar U, Hummer AJ, Nobrega J, Hawkins WG, Coit DG, et al. Cutaneous desmoplastic melanoma: reappraisal of morphologic heterogeneity and prognostic factors. Am J Surg Pathol. 2004;28:1518–25. https://doi.org/10.1097/01.pas.0000141391.91677.a4.
14. Cook MG, Massi D, Szumera-Ciećkiewicz A, Van den Oord J, Blokx W, van Kempen LC, et al. An updated European Organisation for Research and Treatment of Cancer (EORTC) protocol for pathological evaluation of sentinel lymph nodes for melanoma. Eur J Cancer. 2019;114:1–7. https://doi.org/10.1016/j.ejca.2019.03.010.
15. Gershenwald JE, Scolyer RA, Hess KR, Thompson JF, Long GV, Ross MI, et al. Melanoma of the skin. In: Amin MB, Edge SB, Greene FL, et al., editors. AJCC Cancer Staging Manual. 8th ed. New York: Springer; 2017. p. 563–85.

Chapter 2
Basic Medical Physics

Geetha Menon

Radiation therapy for skin cancers involves both external beam radiotherapy (RT) and brachytherapy (BT). The external beam option includes superficial X-rays, orthovoltage X-rays, megavoltage X-rays, or electrons. The choice of the modality, radiation type, and energy depends on tumor geometry: location, depth, volume, and proximity to surrounding critical tissue. Appropriate selection of the modality and delivery technique is dependent on the tumor characteristics and to a large extent on the physics of the radiation beam.

Superficial and Orthovoltage Radiotherapy (SXRT/DXRT)

Superficial (SXRT) and orthovoltage (DXRT) radiotherapy X-ray machines are two low-energy X-ray delivery techniques operating in the kilovoltage range from 50 to 150 kVp and 150 to 300 kVp, respectively. Modern low-energy machines commonly use DXRT, which is an attractive choice for treating skin cancer because of the maximum dose deposition on the skin surface and rapid dose falloff thereafter. Despite advanced treatment deliveries made possible with linear accelerators (linacs), kilovoltage machines are still in use for their quick accessibility, easy setup, and acceptable treatment outcomes.

G. Menon (✉)
Department of Oncology, University of Alberta, Edmonton, AB, Canada

Department of Medical Physics, Cross Cancer Institute, Edmonton, AB, Canada
e-mail: geetha.menon@albertahealthservices.ca

K. J. Joseph et al. (eds.), *Radiotherapy in Skin Cancer*,
https://doi.org/10.1007/978-3-031-44316-9_2

Interaction of Low-Energy Photons with Matter: Photoelectric Effect

The three principal mechanisms of energy deposition by photons in matter are photoelectric effect (PEE), Compton scattering, and pair production. Of these, PEE is the dominant interaction at low photon energies (up to ~0.1 MeV), the energy range where SXRT/DXRT operates [1]. During this process, the incident photon interacts with an inner shell electron, resulting in the complete absorption of the photon and the ejection of the electron (Fig. 2.1).

The energy of the ejected electron (E_e), also called a photoelectron, is given by

$$E_e = E_{ph} - E_b$$

where E_{ph} is the incident photon energy and E_b is the binding energy of the electron shell. The vacancy created by the photoelectron is immediately filled by an electron from an outer orbital followed by the emission of characteristic X-rays with an energy equal to the difference in binding energies of the orbitals.

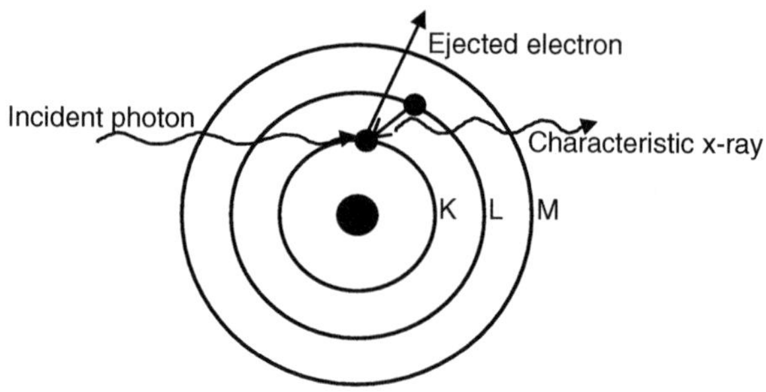

Fig. 2.1 Schematic representation of photoelectric effect. The incident photon interacts with a K-shell electron resulting in the emission of a photoelectron

Energy and Atomic Number Dependence

The probability of PEE occurring is highly dependent on the energy of the incident photon and the atomic number of the attenuator through which it passes. As the incident photon energy increases, the PEE interaction probability decreases. On the other hand, the probability of PEE increases with increasing atomic number. In general, PEE follows a Z^3/E^3 dependence, where Z is the atomic number of the material and E is the incident photon energy (Fig. 2.2). The dependence of the three interaction mechanisms on energy and atomic number is shown in Fig. 2.2. The PEE causes relatively high absorption of energy in bone because of the high atomic number ($Z = 13–14$).

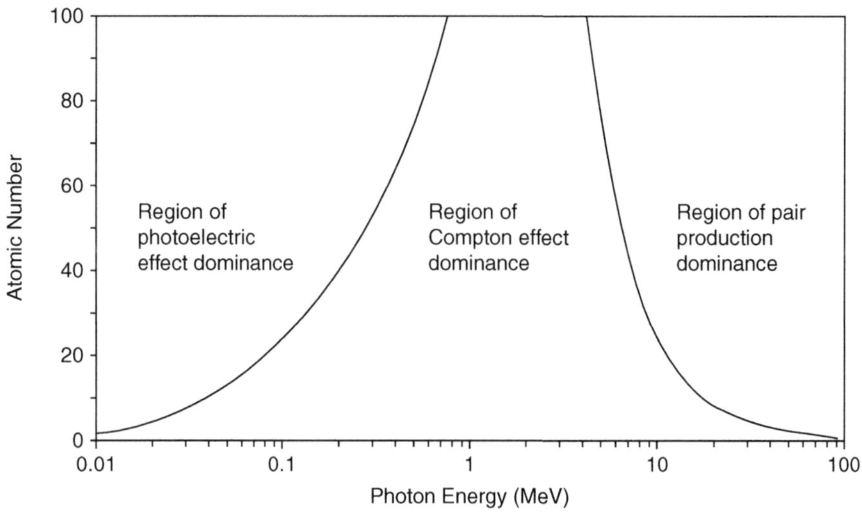

Fig. 2.2 Variation of the three major interaction processes of photons with matter as a function of the atomic number and energy. The energy range over which photoelectric effect, Compton effect, and pair production are dominant is illustrated

Half-Value Layer

Beam quality of low-energy X-ray beams is defined by the half-value layer (HVL), which is the absorber thickness required to attenuate the original beam intensity by half [2]. Typically, appropriate metals of high atomic numbers are used as attenuators or filters to change the beam quality. However, since these filters introduce characteristic X-rays (see previous section) along with the removal of a portion of the lower energy spectrum, composite filters are used.

Composite filters have layers of metals of differential thicknesses and atomic numbers. The metal layers, arranged such that their atomic number decreases away from the X-ray head, preferentially remove the lower photon energies but still retain the original beam intensity [3]. Orthovoltage machines use custom composite filters made from combinations of mainly tin, copper, and aluminum.

Percent Depth Doses

Selection of the SXRT/DXRT energy for treatment is dictated by the penetration depth desired clinically. In this energy range, the maximum dose is deposited on the skin surface and shows a rapid decrease in dose as the depth in the tissue increases, less than 90% at 2 cm depth (Fig. 2.3a) [2]. These machines operate at short focus-to-skin distances (FSD) of either 30 or 50 cm, with field sizes defined by rectangular and circular applicators.

Since the inverse square law effect is a predominant characteristic of SXRT/DXRT beams, the dose rate decreases quadratically with distance, whereby the percent depth dose (PDD) increases with FSD. Consequently, shorter FSD applicators are chosen for superficial lesions, while the longer applicators are preferred for

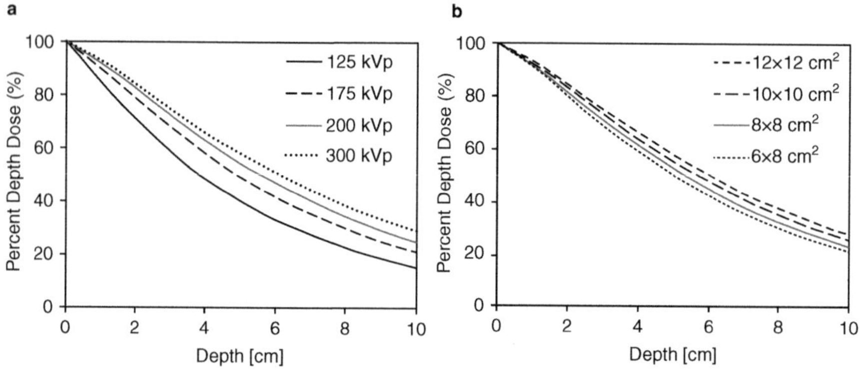

Fig. 2.3 Illustration of percent depth dose curves for a 30 cm focus-to-skin distance orthovoltage applicator (**a**) having a field size of 10×10 cm^2 for energies from 125 to 300 kVp and (**b**) for different field sizes using 200 kVp energy

thicker tumors. For example, consider a superficial tumor of 2 cm depth. If the surface dose is 100%, the dose at 2 cm with a 30 cm FSD applicator will be approximately $(30/30 + 2)^2 = 87.9\%$, while that with a 50 cm FSD would be $(50/50 + 2)^2 = 92.5\%$. Unlike megavoltage photons, orthovoltage X-rays are less forward peaked and affected by higher side scatter, which makes the profiles bulge out at deeper depths in tissue. For the same beam energy, the PDD increases with applicator size due to this increased scatter contribution to the central axis (Fig. 2.3b).

Effect of f-Factor in Superficial/Orthovoltage Treatments

The f-factor is a function of photon energy and the medium. Traditionally, the term f-factor converts radiation exposure in air to absorbed dose in medium and serves as a measure of the attenuation in different medium and hence the absorbed dose. With PEE being the predominant interaction in the kilovoltage energy range, SXRT/DXRT X-rays are significantly influenced by differences in the atomic number of the materials in its path [4]. Presence of high-atomic-number materials, like bone or shields, will enhance dose to adjacent tissue and those upstream from it [5].

The f-factor increases as the beam energy decreases and the atomic number of the medium increases (Fig. 2.4) [6]. For example, in the energy range between 150 and 300 kVp, the f-factor for water ($Z = 7.5$) and muscle ($Z = 7.6$) changes by <0.5%, while that for bone ($Z = 13–14$) differs by ~14% [7]. The f-factor for bone is about fourfold higher at lower energies as the atomic number of bone is much higher compared to water and muscle (13–14 vs. 7–8) (Fig. 2.4) [8]. As Compton interaction probability is dependent on the electron density, which is similar for most tissue, the f-factor is nearly the same for all materials for energies >0.5 MeV [7].

The f-factor variation has a significant impact on the dose when there is bone under soft tissue, a scenario common to SXRT/DXRT treatments. Due to the large

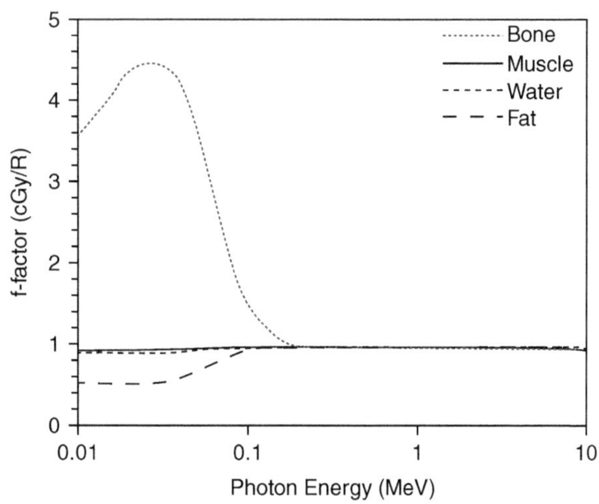

Fig. 2.4 Variation of f-factors for bone, muscle, water, and fat with photon energy. Due to photoelectric effect, the change in f-factor for high atomic number materials, like bone, is significant at low energies

difference in f-factors for bone (1.9) to tissue (0.94) at this beam quality, the dose increase in the bone is twice that in tissue near the interface and subsequently decreases beyond the bone due to increased attenuation [2]. Depending on the beam energy and bone composition, the dose could almost have a fourfold increase.

Field Defining Cutouts and Internal Shields

In SXRT/DXRT, the area to be treated being superficial is clearly identified by a "clinical markup" through visual examination and palpation, with a field margin (1.0–1.5 cm) added to account for any microscopic disease spread. Treatments are usually delivered using an appositional single field with the applicator positioned directly on the tumor to ensure reproducibility in setup for fractionated deliveries.

Cutouts: Custom lead or Cerrobend cutouts are placed on the skin surface to define the beam shape and protect the surrounding normal tissue. Cutouts are designed such that the beam transmission is reduced to no more than 5% transmission of the delivered dose, and for lead, this is >4.32 HVLs (4–5 HVLs) [2]. Generally, 5 mm lead thickness is recommended for 300 kVp and 2 mm for lower energies. With its malleable property, lead cutouts can be easily customized to the geometry of the lesion and conformed to the surface anatomy.

Internal shields: Tissues beyond the treatment depth are affected by exit dose, which can be reduced using internal shields placed behind the treatment region. Examples include the use of tungsten eye shields to reduce lens dose when treating the eyelids and lead oral shields to reduce irradiation of the oral cavity during treatment of the lip. Ideally, the thickness of the shield is selected to reduce transmission to <3%. Thicknesses for both the cutouts and shields should preferably be measured locally for the SXRT/DXRT energies used by the clinic.

Backscatter from the shielding material becomes a concern when using SXRT/DXRT X-rays. The internal shields are coated with wax to absorb these backscattered photons [9]. Similarly, placement of lead cutouts on the skin leads to considerable dose enhancement at the border of the treated and untreated skin. It is recommended that the cutouts be draped in plastic foil wraps to absorb these electrons [10]. On the other hand, in cases where there is lack of backscatter tissue, such as during the treatment of the pinna, there will be a reduction in dose [9].

Surface Heterogeneities: Stand-Off and Stand-In Corrections

In situations of surface inhomogeneities where appositional applicator placement is not possible, the tumor may extend into the applicator (stand-in; increases tumor dose) or be positioned at a distance from the applicator end (stand-off; decreases tumor dose). Inverse square law corrections must be applied to account for the

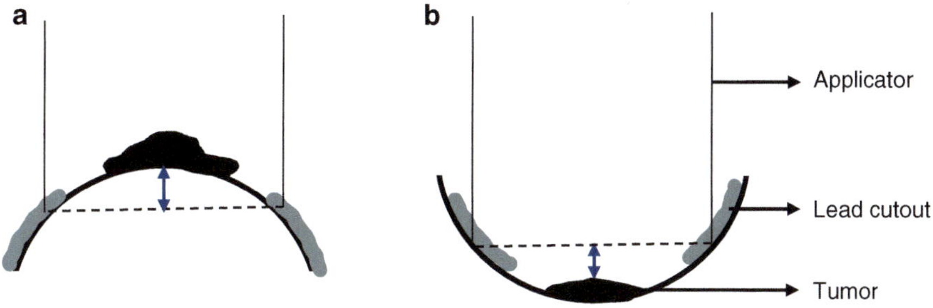

Fig. 2.5 Schematic representation of (**a**) stand-in and (**b**) stand-off when the applicator is not appositionally placed on the skin surface. The blue arrows represent the distance to be used for inverse square law correction when calculating dose

stand-in or stand-off the tumor has with respect to the applicator end (Fig. 2.5). During appositional treatments, care should be taken to avoid ingression by tissue compression, which decreases the FSD and, in turn, increases the surface dose.

Superficial/Orthovoltage Dose Calculation

Clinical dose calculations for orthovoltage treatments are relatively simple as they can be easily performed manually using pre-tabulated data for the different energies and applicators. The factors needed for dose calculation include the applicator dose rate, PDD, and backscatter factors.

Dose rate at the prescription depth ($\dot{D}_{\text{pres}}$) is calculated as

$$\dot{D}_{\text{pres}} = \dot{D}_{\text{appl}} \times \text{PDD} \times \frac{\text{BSF}_{\text{cutout}}}{\text{BSF}_{\text{appl}}} \times \text{ISL},$$

where $\dot{D}_{\text{appl}}$ is the dose rate for the applicator selected, PDD is the percent depth dose for the applicator and energy, $\text{BSF}_{\text{cutout}}$ and BSF_{appl} are the backscatter factors for the cutout and applicator, respectively, and ISL is the inverse square law to account for any stand-off or stand-in.

Electron Beam RT

With the increasing availability of linacs and the suitable characteristics of this radiation, electrons have been replacing SXRT/DXRT as the popular treatment option for skin cancers. The most appealing attribute of electrons for treating superficial lesions is its PDD: deposition of maximum doses closer to the surface and a rapid dose falloff with penetration in tissue, which is desirable for sparing deeper healthy tissue. In addition, the problem of dose enhancement to lesions located above high-atomic-number materials, like bone, due to PEE in orthovoltage treatment can be overcome using electrons.

Electron Percent Depth Dose

Electrons continuously lose energy in small fractions until it comes to rest. When averaged over its entire travel range, the typical energy loss in tissue is about 2 MeV/cm [11]. There are two depths in an electron PDD that are important for treatment planning (Fig. 2.6):

(i) Ideally, for electron treatments, coverage by the 90% isodose line is needed at the posterior or base of the lesion to prevent undertreatment. Hence, understanding of the depth at which the PDD curve falls to 90% (R_{90}; therapeutic range) is important for treatment prescriptions.
(ii) The practical range is the depth of intersection of the steepest portion of the PDD curve and the extrapolation line from the bremsstrahlung tail [11].

Electron beams are contaminated by bremsstrahlung X-rays produced by collision of the electrons with objects in its path such as parts of the accelerator, air between the accelerator head and patient, and the patient itself.

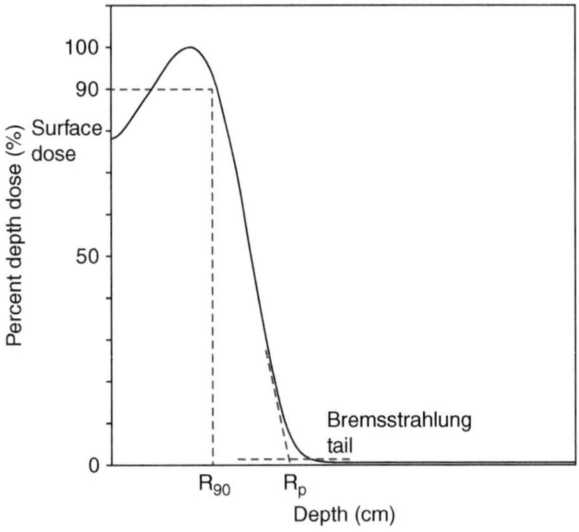

Fig. 2.6 Schematic of a typical electron percent depth dose, showing the surface dose, depth of 90% dose (R_{90}), practical range (R_P), and the Bremsstrahlung tail

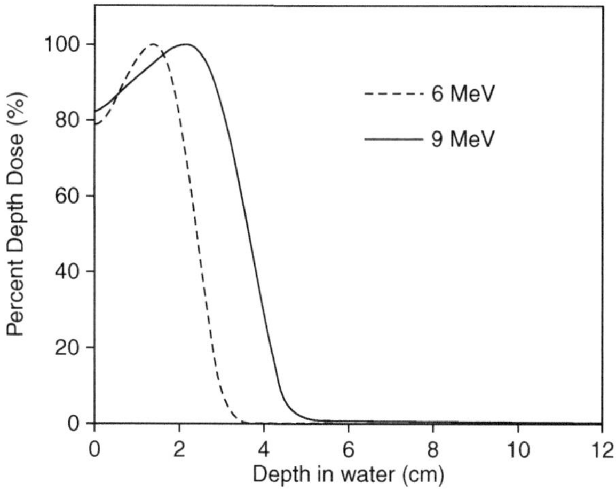

Fig. 2.7 Percent depth dose curves for the 6 and 9 MeV electrons from a high-energy linear accelerator. Typically, these energies are preferred for skin cancer treatment owing to their high skin dose and dramatic falloff after a few centimeters in tissue

A few useful rules of thumb when choosing an electron of energy, E, are [3]:

(i) Percent surface dose $\cong 72 + E$
(ii) Depth of 90% $\cong E/4$
(iii) Range in water $\cong E/2$

Thus, the choice of energy depends on the thickness of the lesion and the depth of desired posterior coverage including the bolus (Fig. 2.7).

Bolus

As seen in Fig. 2.7, the dose at the surface of electron energies used for skin treatments is around 80–90%. Hence, most electron treatments are performed with a bolus to bring the surface dose, where the lesion is, to the maximum. The thickness of the bolus is determined by the depth of maximum dose from the PDD curve of the electron beam. Bolus also helps to smoothen irregular surfaces, which can negatively affect the treatment by introducing pockets of high and low doses. A bolus of differential thickness can even out the surface irregularity and make the dose distribution homogeneous. Electron boluses are made of tissue-equivalent material, wax, and, in modern times, can also be 3D printed.

Electron Field Shaping

Electrons undergo several scattering events after exiting the scattering foil in the linac head, creating a large penumbra not suitable for treatment. To overcome this issue, two levels of collimation are introduced between the linac and the patient surface.

Applicators: Electron applicators or cones are inserted into the head of the linac to collimate the beam and define the field size. These detachable rectangular applicators come in different sizes, typically ranging from 6×6 cm^2 to 25×25 cm^2, and have heights of about 30 cm. The applicator end is placed close to the skin of the patient to decrease electron scatter.

Cutouts: To customize the electron field to irregular shapes, cutouts made of lead or cerrobend are inserted in the rectangular applicator. The cutout thickness is intended to reduce transmission to less than 5%.

Internal shields: As in kilovoltage treatments, for certain electron treatments like that of the buccal mucosa, lip and eyelids, use of internal shields is helpful to protect normal tissue beyond the treatment depth.

Electron Backscatter

The cutouts used for shaping the fields cause electron scatter that changes the output and the beam characteristics such as the depth of maximum dose and penumbra [11]. There can also be significant dose enhancement in tissue near shields due to electron backscatter. When shields are used without being coated with a tissue-equivalent material, such as in the case of internal eye shields, hot spots are observed about 2–3 mm into the eyelid. Hence, to reduce the dose contribution from backscatter electrons, the shields are coated with a low-atomic-number material like wax. It is warranted that individual measurements of the cutouts and shields be performed to understand their dosimetric impact and the corrections be incorporated in the treatment plan.

Effect of Treatment Field Size

As the PDDs and outputs increase with field size and energy, measurements of these factors must be performed for every applicator—energy combination for treatment planning purposes. When the treatment field size is smaller than the practical range of the electron, there is lateral scatter disequilibrium which rapidly decreases the dose rate and shifts the depth of maximum dose closer to the surface (Fig. 2.8). Thus, to define small fields using cutouts for superficial treatments, the size of the field should be at least equal to the electron range necessary for lateral dose buildup. Additionally, specific measurements to determine the output factor should be performed for dose calculations [2].

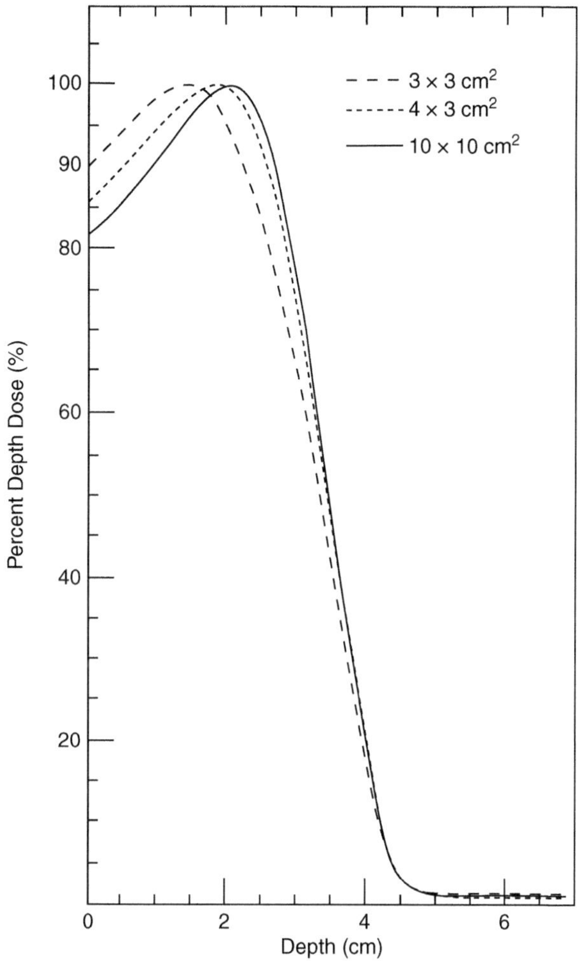

Fig. 2.8 Illustration of the variation in the percent depth dose curves with increasing field sizes of 3 × 3, 4 × 4, and 10 × 10 cm^2 for a 9 MeV electron beam

Isodose Profile Characteristics

Isodose profiles of low-energy electron beams used in superficial treatments have a slight lateral constriction of the higher isodoses on the surface (Fig. 2.9). This necessitates the need for defining appropriate margins (at least 1.0–1.5 cm) around the tumor bed to avoid underdosing at depth. Furthermore, the isodoses show a lateral bulge with depth due to increased electron scattering in the medium. This is of concern when using abutted electron fields for treatment where the lower isodose curves will spread to the adjacent field; however, for skin treatments, such field placements are not commonly used.

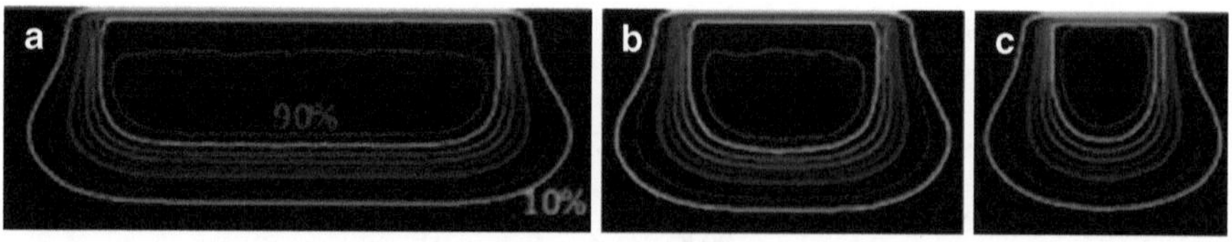

Fig. 2.9 Isodose profiles for a 9 MeV electron beam using a (**a**) 10 × 10, (**b**) 5 × 5, and (**c**) 3 × 3 cm^2 field size and a source-to-surface distance of 100 cm

Effect of Inhomogeneities

Penetration depth of electrons is dependent on the electron density, which is same for most tissues in the human body. Electron treatments are delivered standardly using a source-to-surface distance (SSD) of 100 cm. The electron applicator end is typically at 95 cm, making a 5 cm gap between the cone end and skin. When this gap is increased, the dose rate decreases and the low isodoses diverge out while the higher isodoses converge to the middle, producing a broader penumbra [7]. Similarly, air gaps between bolus and the patient's skin can also decrease the dose rate. Compared to air, the bolus scatters electrons at wider angles such that fewer electrons will reach a given point on the patient skin surface.

Effects of Beam Obliquity

Generally, electron treatments for skin lesions are delivered using a single head-on field. However, surface inhomogeneities can necessitate the need for using an oblique beam. As the angle of incidence of the beam with the surface increases, the depth of dose maximum and PDD gets shifted towards the surface, i.e., to shallower depths. Due to the increased electron fluence along the central axis of oblique beams, the dose at depth of dose maximum increases significantly; for example, this can be as large as 23% at an angle of 75° for a 9 MeV electron beam [11].

On the other hand, increasing obliquity decreases dose to deeper tissue. Boluses are often used to flatten out irregular surfaces and improve dose homogeneity. In short, angled treatments can have a significant impact on skin cancer treatments with electrons.

Electron Dose Calculation

Though often planned using manual markup, electron treatments benefit from the traditional planning technique of using a CT scan for accurate delineation of the tumor. Modern commercial treatment planning systems are equipped to perform

Table 2.1 Differences in the use of DXRT and electrons for skin cancer treatments

	Orthovoltage	Electrons
Identification of treatment area	Clinical markup	Clinical markup or CT imaging
Margins used	1.0–1.5 cm	At least 1.5 cm
Energies used	150–300 kVp	6 or 9 MeV
F-factor dependence	Large influence of f-factor	No f-factor dependence
Choice of energy	Lesion covered at least by 90% at depth	90% isodose to cover the lesion at depth
Collimator choice	Shorter FSD (30 cm) collimators for superficial lesions and longer FSDs (50 cm) for deeper lesions	All collimators are of the same length
Bolus	100% dose on surface; hence, no bolus	Bolus thickness based on electron energy
Collimation	Size of lesion + margin; shape of applicator	Applicator size and field shaping accessory
External shielding	Custom lead cutouts placed on skin; thickness of cutout is based on DXRT energy	Custom cutouts supported on the electron applicator; output factors of cutouts need to be measured
Internal shielding	Lead or tungsten coated with wax or acrylic	Lead or tungsten coated with wax or acrylic
Dose calculation	Mostly manual	Computerized; using dedicated algorithms
Advantages	Dose maximum on surface Sharper penumbra; simple machine involving easy setup and treatment	Sharp dose falloff, hence more sparing of normal tissue beyond the treatment depth

electron dose calculation using pre-measured data. However, electron beams of the same energy on different linacs will not be the same due to inherent differences in the design. Hence, care should be taken in the selection of treatment data and accompanying parameters, such as cutout factors, for each machine.

In summary, external beam treatments for skin lesions using either orthovoltage or electrons are complex and require thorough knowledge of the physics issues that need to be considered during treatment planning (Table 2.1). Advanced delivery techniques such as IMRT/VMAT are now available on modern linacs and have facilitated the use of high-energy photons for many skin cancers. Brachytherapy is also a competing modality for treating superficial cancers.

References

1. Attix FH. Introduction to radiological physics and radiation dosimetry. New York: J. Wiley and Sons; 1986.
2. Gibbons JP. Khan's the physics of radiation therapy. 6th ed. Philadelphia: Lippincott Williams & Wilkins; 2020.

3. Mayles P, Nahum AE, Rosenwald, J.C. (Eds.). Handbook of radiotherapy physics: theory and practice. 2nd ed. CRC Press; 2021.
4. Papanikolaou N, Battista JJ, Boyer AL, Kappas C, Klein E, Mackie TR, Sharpe M, Van Dyk J. Tissue inhomogeneity corrections for megavoltage photon beams. AAPM Task Group. 2004;65:1.
5. Huq MS, Venkataramanan N, Meli JA. The effect on dose of kilovoltage x-rays backscattered from lead. Int J Radiat Oncol Biol Phys. 1992;24(1):171–5.
6. Seuntjens J, Thierens H, Van der Plaetsen A, Segaert O. Conversion factor f for X-ray beam qualities, specified by peak tube potential and HVL value. Phys Med Biol. 1987;32(5):595–603.
7. Johns HE, Cunningham JR. The physics of radiology. 4th ed. Charles C. Thomas; 1983.
8. Tepper JE, Foote RL, Michalski JM. Gunderson & Tepper's clinical radiation oncology. 5th ed. Philadelphia: Elsevier; 2021.
9. Eaton DJ, Doolan PJ. Review of backscatter measurement in kilovoltage radiotherapy using novel detectors and reduction from lack of underlying scattering material. J Appl Clin Med Phys. 2013;14(6):4358.
10. Lye JE, Butler DJ, Webb DV. Enhanced epidermal dose caused by localized electron contamination from lead cutouts used in kilovoltage radiotherapy. Med Phys. 2010;37(8):3935–9.
11. Podgorsak EB. Radiation oncology physics: a handbook for teachers and students. International Atomic Energy Agency Publication; 2005.

Chapter 3
Skin Radiotherapy Treatment Planning

Arun Elangovan, Beena Kunheri, and Kurian Jones Joseph

General Considerations

Patient Selection

Radiotherapy (RT) is offered either as a primary or as an adjuvant therapy for skin cancers. RT is commonly recommended for elderly patients with comorbidities, those who decline surgery, and especially for lesions around the eyelids, external ear, nose, eyebrows, or lips where primary surgery could result in significant cosmetic or functional deficits. Radiotherapy alone provides local control rates ranging from 85 to 100% and generally preserves the tissue anatomy and functions [1, 2]. However, RT may be contraindicated in patients with:

- Associated radiosensitive conditions like xeroderma pigmentosum, basal cell nevus syndrome, or Gorlin's syndrome
- Scleroderma
- Other connective tissue diseases such as SLE in active phase

A. Elangovan
Division of Radiation Oncology, Cross Cancer Institute, Edmonton, AB, Canada

B. Kunheri
Hamad Medical Corporation, National Center for Cancer Care and Research (NCCCR), Doha, Qatar

K. J. Joseph (✉)
Division of Radiation Oncology, Cross Cancer Institute, & Department of Oncology, University of Alberta, Edmonton, AB, Canada
e-mail: kurian.joseph@albertahealthservices.ca

K. J. Joseph et al. (eds.), *Radiotherapy in Skin Cancer*,
https://doi.org/10.1007/978-3-031-44316-9_3

Relative contraindications to RT include:

- Young age
- Previously irradiated site, depending on various factors
- Poorly vascularized areas, e.g., back of elbow, front of knee, and lower leg
- Hair-bearing skin, when permanent alopecia is a concern

Tumor Factors

Tumor characteristics including the histology, size, and location are critical determinants of the actual target volume to be treated and the RT technique to be chosen.

Squamous cell carcinoma (SCC) or basal cell carcinoma (BCC) of the skin with high-risk features can be associated with high rates of local recurrence from 20% to 50% with surgery alone, and postoperative RT is often recommended to optimize locoregional control [3]. General indications are patients with:

- T3/T4 disease
- Positive or inadequate surgical margins
- Perineural invasion (PNI)

Patients with T2 disease and associated with one or more of the following risk factors:

- Poor differentiation
- Depth/thickness >4 mm or infiltration deeper to subcutaneous fat
- Desmoplastic or infiltrative growth pattern with immunosuppressed status
- Recurrent lesions
- Lesions at the ear and hair-bearing lip/vermillion lip
- Microscopic PNI
- Lymphovascular space invasion (LVI)
- Immunosuppressed status

Steps Involved in Treatment Planning

Once a patient has decided to proceed with RT, a step-by-step approach is recommended for treatment planning and delivery. In general, smaller lesions are treated with either superficial RT (SXRT), orthovoltage RT (DXRT), or electrons (6–9 MeV with bolus), and large or locally advanced tumors are treated with high-energy electrons (9–12 MeV) or megavoltage photons, most often, but not always, as an adjuvant therapy. Treatments using brachytherapy are described in Chap. 15.

The steps in external RT planning include the following:

Target Volume Definition

Target volume definition is the key to decide whether a patient will be best treated with either SXRT/DXRT, electrons, or high-energy photons. Target volume definition is mainly based on clinical examination.

Gross Tumor Volume (GTV)

- For small tumors, GTV can often be defined by clinical examination alone. Magnifying glass may be used for precise target delineation, and the tumor extent can be marked directly on the skin surface.
- For large or locally advanced lesions, or when local invasion into the adjacent structures or lymph nodal involvement is suspected, computed tomography (CT) or magnetic resonance imaging (MRI) should be considered for target definition.

Clinical Target Volume (CTV)

The CTV is defined after precise assessment of the tumor spread and based on the proximity of tumor to adjacent normal tissues/organs at risk (OAR). CTV encompasses all the microscopic extent of disease, and this requires estimation of a safety margin around the visible edge of the tumor. This margin depends on:

- Tumor size
- Histology
- Perineural invasion
- Tumor thickness
- Location and proximity to OARs

Typically, a CTV margin of 0.5–1 cm is used for small well-defined BCC with a visible tumor edge, and a margin of 1–2 cm is recommended for poorly defined or large infiltrative lesions. Khan et al. prospectively defined the required CTV margin for SCC and BCC to minimize the risk of local recurrence [4]. The study noted that the microscopic tumor extent positively correlated with the size of the gross lesion, tumor histology, and number of surgical attempts that were required to obtain a clear margin. The CTV recommendations to provide a 95% or greater chance of covering microscopic disease were defined to be:

- 10 mm for BCC less than 2 cm and 13 mm for BCC greater than 2 cm
- 11 mm for SCC less than 2 cm and 14 mm for SCC greater than 2 cm

Geographical miss is the most common cause of treatment failure following skin RT. Hence, it is critical to determine the extent of tumor infiltration into the deeper tissues and fixation to the surrounding structures to appropriately define the

CTV. Skin lesions originating at embryonal fusion planes are particularly at greater risk of deep invasion, and therefore, lesions located at the inner canthus of eye, philtrum, chin, nasolabial groove, and preauricular and retro-auricular regions should be meticulously evaluated for appropriate inclusion of the subclinical microscopic disease within the target volume.

Optimal management of possible subclinical PNI along the nerve trunk observed either clinically or radiologically is less well defined, although expert recommendations favor treatment of PNI in head and neck cutaneous SCC and BCC with inclusion of the entire cranial nerve trunk up to the skull base within the CTV [5, 6]. This would almost always require conformal planning using intensity-modulated radiation techniques for precise target definition and dose delivery. Elective treatment of possible PNI involving peripheral nerves in cases of cutaneous cancers of the extremities is impractical and is of unproven benefit.

Planning Target Volume (PTV)

PTV is the margin around CTV, primarily includes a margin for day-to-day setup variations, and is dependent on the treatment technique and beam energy. A minimum margin of 3–5 mm may be adequate, depending on the RT modality (Fig. 3.1).

Selection of RT Technique

The decision to use a specific treatment technique depends on the following:

- **Tumor size**: In general, smaller lesions are treated with either SXRT/DXRT or electrons, and large or locally advanced tumors are treated with higher energy electrons or megavoltage photons, most often as an adjuvant therapy.

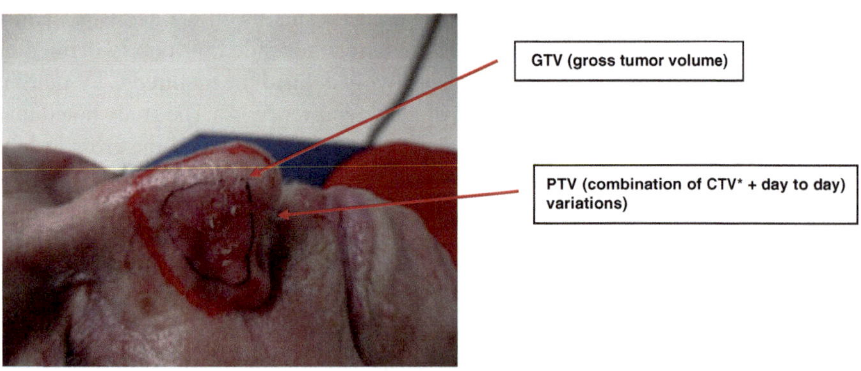

Fig. 3.1 An 80-year-old patient with basal cell carcinoma involving the right ala of nose. Gross tumor volume, GTV (black), and planning target volume, PTV (red), are marked. **CTV* Clinical target volume

- **Anatomical location of the tumor**: Small tumors on the face are preferably treated with SXRT or DXRT, and those overlying the bone are commonly treated with electrons.
- **Adjacent OAR**: It is vital to understand tumor relations to the surrounding structures (e.g., bone, air cavities) due to differences in radiobiological interactions observed with the different RT modalities. At lower photon energies, X-rays interact with matter primarily via the photoelectric effect (PEE). PEE depends on the atomic number (Z) of the absorbing material and the photon energy (E) (PEE α Z^3/E^3). This causes a relatively high absorption of energy in bone. This differential absorption is described in terms of f-factor, which relates exposure of radiation in air to the absorbed dose of radiation in tissue. Bone has a comparatively high atomic number, and for energies below 250 kVp, the f-factor for bone is $\geq$4 times the f-factors for water and tissue [7]. This results in increased dose absorption in the bone compared to the surrounding tissue. As the atomic numbers of water and tissue are similar to that of air, their f-factors do not vary much over the range of energies. Hence, for tissues overlying bony structures, either electron or megavoltage photon therapy is preferred.
- **Tumor thickness:** Assessing tumor thickness and the extent of deep tissue infiltration is essential to determine the prescription depth and for selection of the preferred RT modality.

Superficial or Orthovoltage Irradiation

SXRT or DXRT is the preferred treatment for small and superficial tumors [8]. The treatment planning process with SXRT/DXRT is generally referred to as "clinical markup." The markup section involves a radiation oncologist, a medical physicist, and a radiation therapist. Once the lesion to be treated is assessed, the GTV is marked around the lesion on the skin surface, and in routine clinical practice, an additional margin around the GTV is provided that includes both CTV and PTV (Fig. 3.1). Field customization is then achieved with lead cutouts placed on the patient's skin. The targets (GTV and PTV) marked on the skin surface can then be traced on to a transparency sheet (Fig. 3.2) that would help to check the daily target position before RT and to minimize day-to-day setup variations.

Once PTV is defined, appropriate beam energy is chosen so that the depth of PTV is covered by 85–90% isodose. In general, 100 kVp would be suitable for lesions measuring no more than 3–4 mm in depth. Most of the uncomplicated cases can be treated to a depth of 10 mm with 150 kVp (85% dose to cover PTV). For thicker lesions and lip cancers, higher energies in the order of 200 kVp are needed to treat a depth of 1.2 cm (85% dose) and 300 kVp to adequately cover a depth of 1.5 cm (90% dose) (Fig. 3.3). Once the beam energy is decided, dose will be prescribed at the skin surface (where 100% dose will be delivered), and the maximum dose is deposited on the surface of the target. Hence, bolus is not required for a dose buildup while using SXRT or DXRT [9].

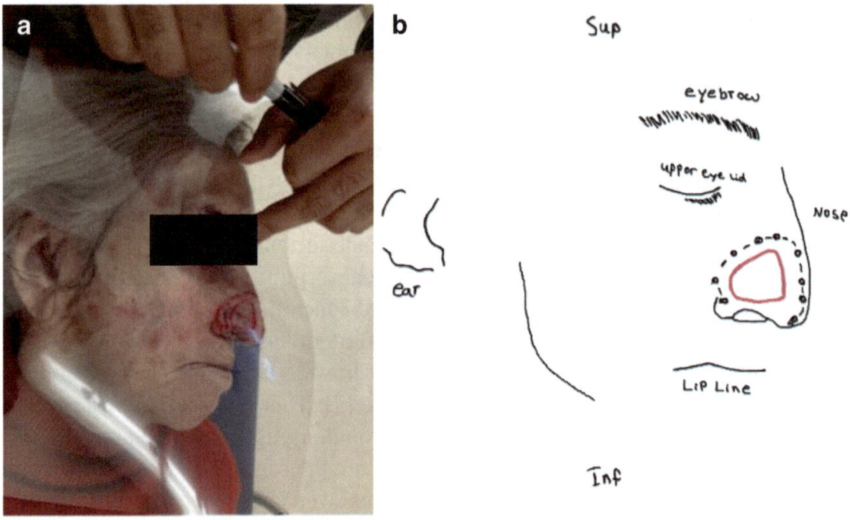

Fig. 3.2 (**a**, **b**) An example of lesion tracing onto a transparency sheet

Typically, patient immobilization or simulation CT scans are not required for SXRT/DXRT planning. Simple and comfortable patient positioning using head rings or neck supports is sufficient for reproducing the setup, depending on the site to be treated.

Applicators of various sizes and shapes (circular, square, or rectangular) are available to direct SXRT/DXRT. Table 3.1 provides a common list of applicators used. Selection of the applicator is based on the size and shape of the target, as well as the location of the tumor. Percentage depth dose (PDD) varies significantly as a function of beam energy, skin-to-surface distance (SSD), and field size, and this must be provided to the medical physicist to decide the suitable applicator that would adequately cover the target (Fig. 3.4).

Field customization is achieved with lead cutouts placed on the patient's skin surface to shape the field and to protect the surrounding normal tissues. In general, each RT department keeps a record of the thickness of lead cutouts required for the different kilovoltage energies available. Table 3.2 provides the list of energies available in our department with the required lead thickness. These "entrance shields" are designed such that no more than 3–5% of the transmission of the prescribed dose is allowed to pass through the shielding; this is typically achieved with a thickness of 2–5 mm lead [9]. While preparing a lead cutout, it should be ensured that the lead sheet selected has at least 3 cm of lead beyond the edge of clinical markings. The applicator edge will need to be at least 1 cm from the cutout opening edge, and there needs to be at least 2 cm of lead beyond the edge of the applicator (Fig. 3.5).

The high atomic number of lead results in effective shielding with minimal thickness; however, it is also responsible for dose enhancement at the edge of the treatment field at shallow depths due to photoelectrons generated in the lead (Fig. 3.6).

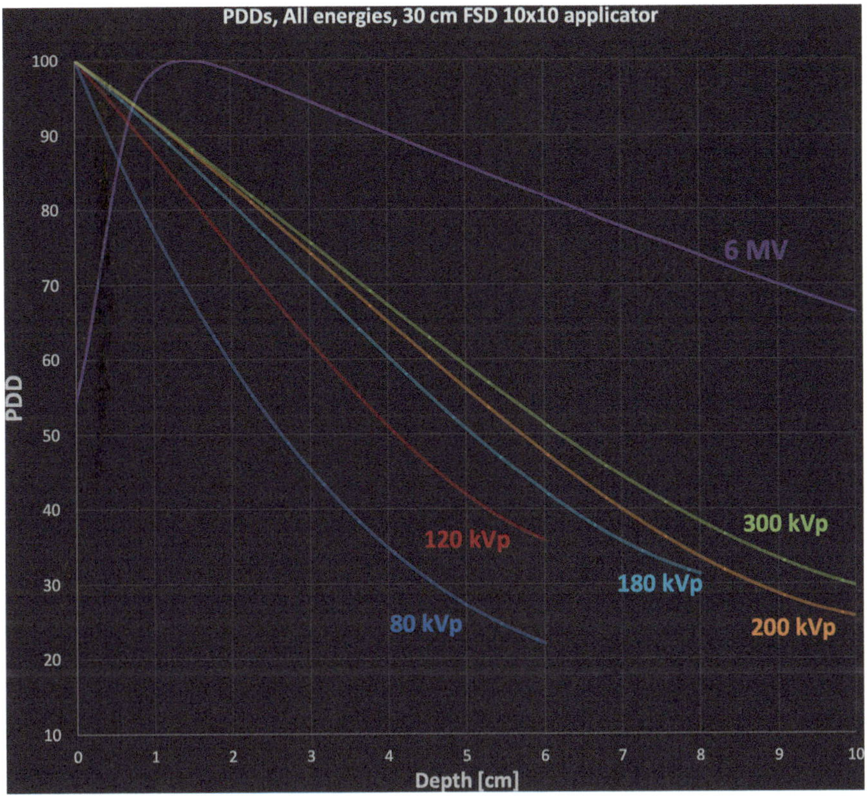

Fig. 3.3 Depth dose curves of common SXRT/DXRT (alongside a 100 cm SSD 6MV photon beam for comparison). The 90% depth dose is at 9 mm for 120 kVp, 11 mm for 180 kVp, and 12–14 mm for 200 and 300 kVp. The surface dose for 6 MV photon is 55%, and 100% dose is at a depth of 15 mm (courtesy of Dr. Lesley Baldwin, Senior Medical Physicist, BC Cancer Agency, Victoria)

Table 3.1 Common list of applicators used for kilovoltage radiotherapy

	Rectangular	
Circular (30 cm SSD)	30 cm SSD	50 cm SSD
3.0	4 × 6	
3.5	6 × 8	6 × 8
4.0	8 × 8	
5.0	8 × 10	8 × 10
6.0	10 × 10	
8.0	12 × 12	10 × 15

This could result in erythema and hyperpigmentation at the junction of treated and untreated skin, leading to poor cosmetic outcomes [10]. The edge dose is enhanced by approximately two- and threefold, respectively, for 150 and 300 kVp beams.

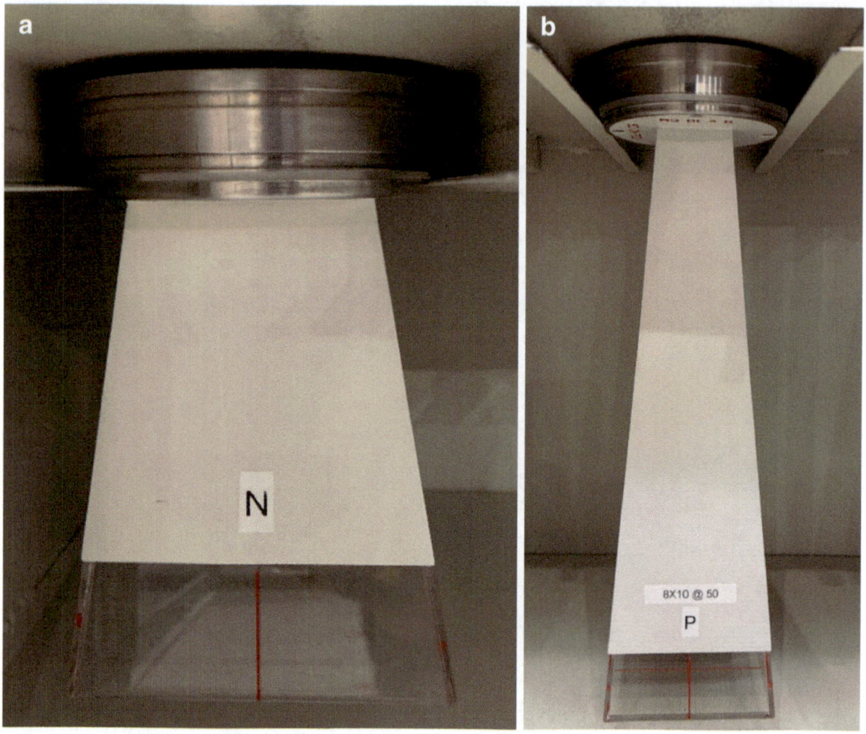

Fig. 3.4 Picture (**a**) shows a 12 × 12 cm square applicator at 30 cm SSD, and picture (**b**) 8 × 10 cm rectangular shows applicator at 50 cm SSD

Table 3.2 Thickness of lead cutouts used in orthovoltage radiotherapy

Energy (kVp)	Lead thickness
80	2 mm
120	
180	
200	
300	5 mm

Plastic films such as Glad Wrap™ or Saran Wrap shielding placed around the lead cutout is a simple way to remove the electron contamination. The thickness of Saran Wrap is decided based on the chosen beam energy. For 300 kVp, ten layers would be needed (each ~200 microns thick), and for 200 kVp, six such layers may be adequate (Fig. 3.6).

Custom shielding may also be done to protect the underlying normal tissues from exit dose (exit dose shielding/internal shielding). The common sites where exit dose shields are used include behind the ear, inside the nostrils, or inside the mouth. Typically, lead shields are used for this purpose. However, backscatter photons from the open field may increase the dose under the shield. This may be critical for eye

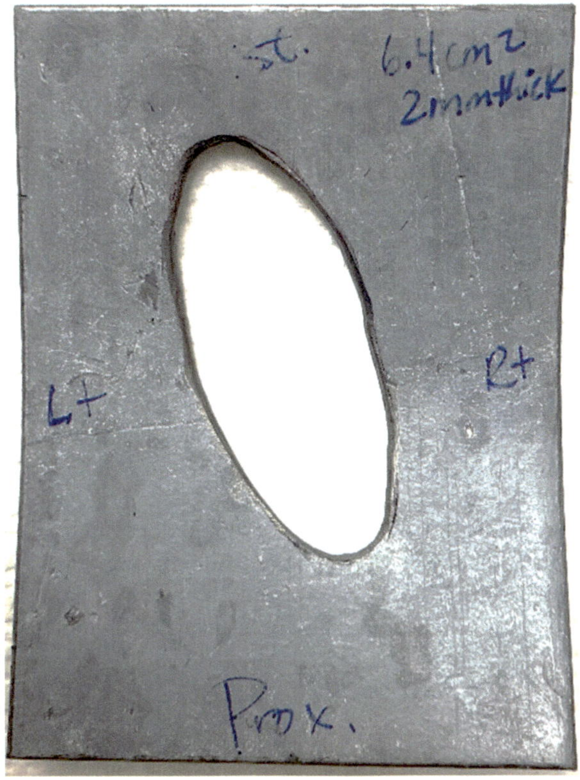

Fig. 3.5 An example of a custom lead cutout used for orthovoltage radiation field shaping

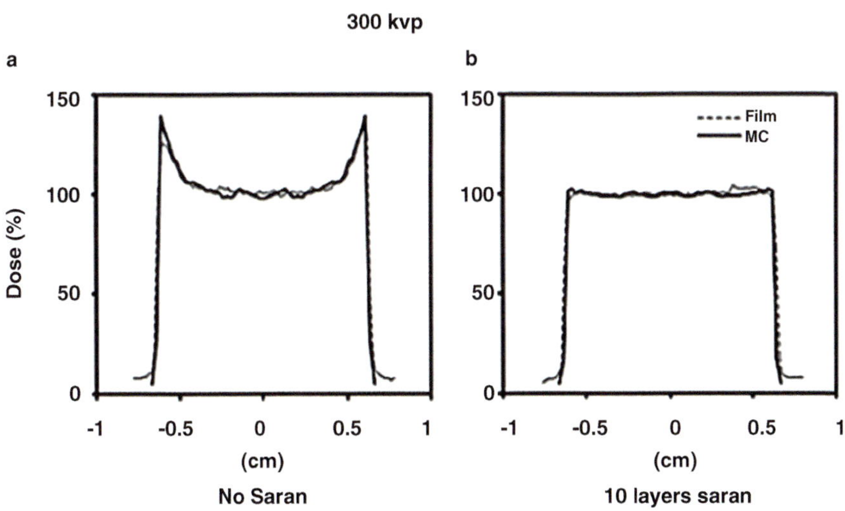

Fig. 3.6 Edge dose enhancement effect with and without plastic wrap shielding around the lead cutout. (**a**) The dose at edges is about 1.4 times central dose (40% enhancement). (**b**) With ten layers of the plastic wrap (~200 microns thick), dose enhancement is corrected (with permission from Lye et al.)

shields and in shields placed adjacent to mucous membranes. To prevent this backscatter from causing toxicities, these shields are coated with wax of varying thickness (depending on the treatment energy chosen) to absorb the backscatter dose [11].

In summary, the unique advantages of orthovoltage RT include:

- Maximum dose on the skin surface
- Narrow penumbra
- Easy setup
- Ease of field shaping with lead cutout

Electron Beam Therapy

Electrons are often used to treat skin lesions over sites like the scalp and superficial to bone or cartilage, where treatment with DXRT may result in excessive bone and cartilaginous dose due to f-factor effect. In general, patients selected for electron beam RT routinely undergo CT simulation. Clinical markup may be performed. For patients who undergo CT simulation, the region of interest should be immobilized to improve treatment reproducibility and to minimize day-to-day setup variations. As skin cancers are usually superficial and are not readily appreciated on CT imaging, the lesion to be treated should be lead-wired before CT simulation to visualize the lesion in CT scan (Fig. 3.7a, b).

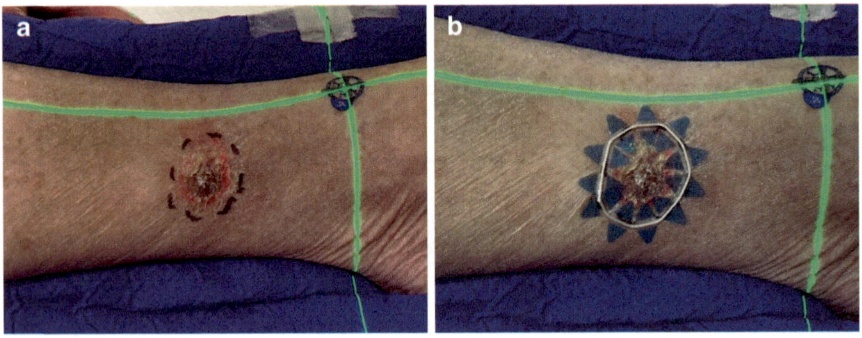

Fig. 3.7 (**a**) 78-Year-old patient with a 2.6 cm biopsy-confirmed squamous cell carcinoma involving the left leg. The limb is appropriately immobilized in a vac-bag. (**b**) The lesion is defined with a lead wire

Planning Considerations for Electron Beam Therapy

Electron beams in tissue typically have a buildup region followed by a Dmax (point of maximum dose along the central axis of the beam), and the dose falls off sharply (2 Mev/cm of water or soft tissue) beyond the 80% maximum dose. Due to the initial buildup, surface dose is only modest, ranging between 75% and 95%. Due to the rapid dose falloff, deeper healthy tissues are significantly spared from toxicities. However, it is also important to ensure that the maximum depth of PTV is adequately encompassed by at least 90% isodose to prevent underdosing the target [12].

After clinical markup, the beam energy is chosen so that the maximum depth of PTV is covered by 90% isodose. The depth of 80% and 90% isodoses (in cm) for a given beam energy (E) can be obtained using the rule of thumb formula D90% ~ E/4 and D80% ~ E/3 [12]. In case of CT planning, dose coverage can be optimized to encompass the tumor depth with the desired target isodose.

When electron beams hit a target, the lower dose isodose curves expand rapidly below the medium due to scattering, and the higher dose isodose curves tend to show lateral constriction at depth, which is worse with smaller fields. Hence, electrons are not preferred as the primary treatment for field sizes smaller than 4 × 4 cm [12] (Fig. 3.8).

As with SXRT/DXRT, electron beam therapy for skin cancers is delivered as a single direct field. Specifically, oblique beam incidences may significantly alter the PDD and should therefore be avoided. The nominal SSD is 100 cm, and the air gap (separation between patient surface and the end of applicator cone) is usually fixed at 5 cm.

Field shaping can be achieved with external shields for irregular targets using lead blocks or cerrobend attached to the end of the applicator cone. Custom shielding for smaller fields may affect the PDD significantly due to decrease in dose contribution from lateral scatter. A lead thickness of 1 mm for every 2 MeV increase in electron energy would be required, in addition to a fixed 1 mm thickness as a safety margin (e.g., 4.5 mm + 1 mm = 5.5 mm for 9 MeV electron beam). Internal shields (coated with wax to prevent backscatter) can be used as appropriate, as in the treatment of eyelid, lip, buccal mucosa, etc. [13].

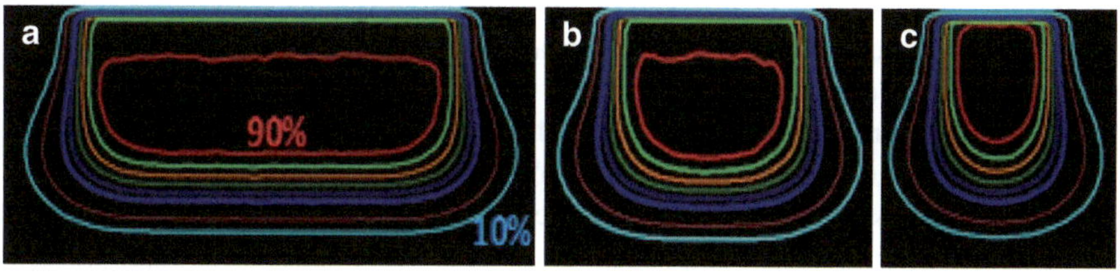

Fig. 3.8 Isodose distributions of a 9 MeV electron beam for (**a**) 10 × 10 cm, (**b**) 5 × 5 cm, and (**c**) 3 × 3 cm field dimensions demonstrating expansion and constriction of isodose curves (courtesy of Dr. Geetha Menon, Medical Physics Dept., Cross Cancer Institute)

Electrons provide a skin-sparing effect, and the entrance dose varies according to beam energy, field size, SSD, and beam obliquity. To achieve a full dose on the surface, a tissue equivalent material such as superflab, custom-made wax, or 3D printed bolus has to be placed on the skin [14]. Bolus may also be used to flatten out irregular surfaces to prevent "stand-off" effect and as tissue compensators.

The unique advantages of electron beams include the following:

- No "f"-factor effect, and hence, dose absorption is not enhanced over bone or cartilage.
- Rapid dose falloff minimizes dose deposition at depths beyond the target volume, resulting in significant sparing of the underlying normal tissues.

Megavoltage photons are used to treat patients with larger lesions or those requiring adjuvant therapy, especially in the head and neck region. Treatment planning is essentially similar to primary head and neck cancer [15].

Treatment Scheme

For SXRT and DXRT, dose will be prescribed at the skin surface (where 100% dose will be delivered), so that target volume is encompassed by the 90% depth dose. In case of electron RT, 100% dose is prescribed to the ICRU reference point so that 90% isodose line covers the PTV. The location of this point should always be at the center or in the central part of the PTV. The beam energy should be selected so that the maximum of the depth-dose curve on the beam axis is located at the center of the PTV.

The relative biological effectiveness (RBE) of electrons is considered to be 10% lower than RBE of kilovoltage beams, and hence, in the past, the dose was specified at 90% isodose to adjust for the lower RBE. However, ICRU 71 reports that no adjustments are needed for dose prescription due to the differences in RBE between photons and electrons but recommends reporting the maximum and minimum doses to the PTV and OARs for all electron beam treatments [16, 17].

Details regarding dose fractionation are described in the chapter on dose fractionation (Chap. 4). In general, fractionation schedules approximately equal a BED_3 of 100 Gy [18]. Several factors should be considered to decide the dose fractionation for each case. Dose fractionation is based on the target volume and OARs that would be included in the treatment field. Hypofractionated regimens are used to treat smaller volumes, and more protracted dose fractionation schedules are generally used for larger treatment targets to minimize late toxicities and to optimize functional and cosmetic outcomes. However, patient factors such as age and performance status should also be considered. We advise caution in the use of large single doses for radical intent treatment. Typically, treatments at 2–2.5 Gy per fraction are delivered to a total dose of 55–60 Gy. For adjuvant treatments, 50 Gy in 20–25 fractions over 4–5 weeks is recommended. For patients with high-risk features, treatments should be planned similar to primary head and neck tumors [19].

References

1. Locke J, Karimpour S, Young G, Lockett MA, Perez CA. Radiotherapy for epithelial skin cancer. Int J Radiat Oncol Biol Phys. 2001;51(3):748–55.
2. Kwan W, Wilson D, Moravan V. Radiotherapy for locally advanced basal cell and squamous cell carcinomas of the skin. Int J Radiat Oncol Biol Phys. 2004;60(2):406–11.
3. Jennings L, Schmults CD. Management of high-risk cutaneous squamous cell carcinoma. J Clin Aesthetic Dermat. 2010;3(4):39–48.
4. Khan L, Choo R, Breen D, Assaad D, Fialkov J, Antonyshyn O, et al. Recommendations for CTV margins in radiotherapy planning for non melanoma skin cancer. Radiother Oncol. 2012;104(2):263–6.
5. Gluck I, Ibrahim M, Popovtzer A, Teknos TN, Chepeha DB, Prince ME, et al. Skin cancer of the head and neck with Perineural invasion: defining the clinical target volumes based on the pattern of failure. Int J Radiat Oncol Biol Phys. 2009;74(1):38–46.
6. Bakst RL, Glastonbury CM, Parvathaneni U, Katabi N, Hu KS, Yom SS. Perineural invasion and perineural tumor spread in head and neck cancer. Int J Radiat Oncol Biol Phys. 2019;103(5):1109–24.
7. Atherton P, Townley J, Glaholm J. Cartilage: the 'F'-factor fallacy. Clin Oncol. 1993;5(6):391–2.
8. McGregor S, Minni J, Herold D. Superficial radiation therapy for the treatment of nonmelanoma skin cancers. J Clin Aesthetic Dermatol. 2015;8(12):12–4.
9. Gerig L, Soubra M, Salhani D. Beam characteristics of the Therapax DXT300 orthovoltage therapy unit. Phys Med Biol. 1994;39(9):1377–92.
10. Lye JE, Butler DJ, Webb DV. Enhanced epidermal dose caused by localized electron contamination from lead cutouts used in kilovoltage radiotherapy. Med Phys. 2010;37(8):3935–9.
11. Das IJ, Chopra KL. Backscatter dose perturbation in kilovoltage photon beams at high atomic number interfaces. Med Phys. 1995;22(6):767–73.
12. Hogstrom KR, Almond PR. Review of electron beam therapy physics. Phys Med Biol. 2006;51(13):R455–89.
13. Shiu AS, Tung SS, Gastorf RJ, Hogstrom KR, Morrison WH, Peters LJ. Dosimetric evaluation of lead and tungsten eye shields in electron beam treatment. Int J Radiat Oncol Biol Phys. 1996;35(3):599–604.
14. Low DA, Starkschall G, Buinowski SW, Wang LL, Hogstrom KR. Electron bolus Design for Radiotherapy Treatment Planning: bolus design algorithms. Med Phys. 1992;19(1):115–24.
15. Gupta T, Sinha S, Ghosh-Laskar S, Budrukkar A, Mummudi N, Swain M, et al. Intensity-modulated radiation therapy versus three-dimensional conformal radiotherapy in head and neck squamous cell carcinoma: long-term and mature outcomes of a prospective randomized trial. Radiat Oncol. 2020;15(1):218.
16. Gahbauer R, Landberg T, Chavaudra J, Dobbs J, Gupta N, Hanks G, et al. Prescribing, recording, and reporting electron beam therapy. J ICRU. 2004;4:1.
17. Berthelsen AK, Dobbs J, Kjellén E, Landberg T, Möller TR, Nilsson P, et al. What's new in target volume definition for radiologists in ICRU report 71? How can the ICRU volume definitions be integrated in clinical practice? Cancer Imaging. 2007;7:104.
18. Zaorsky NG, Lee CT, Zhang E, Keith SW, Galloway TJ. Hypofractionated radiation therapy for basal and squamous cell skin cancer: a meta-analysis. Radiother Oncol. 2017;125(1):13–20.
19. Likhacheva A, Awan M, Barker CA, Bhatnagar A, Bradfield L, Brady MS, et al. Definitive and postoperative radiation therapy for basal and squamous cell cancers of the skin: executive summary of an American Society for Radiation Oncology clinical practice guideline. Pract Radiat Oncol. 2020;10(1):8–20.

Chapter 4
Dose Fractionation in Skin Radiotherapy

Winkle Kwan

Standard Once-a-Day Fractionations

Publications on the efficacy and safety of radiotherapy in the treatment of non-melanoma skin cancers (NMSCs) tend to utilize a potpourri of dose fractionations. In general, smaller tumors were treated with shorter regimens, whereas larger tumors were treated with longer dose fractionations. This reflects our knowledge of how late effects of radiotherapy depend on both dose per fraction and volume of tissue treated. From these publications, particularly older ones in which a wider variety of dose per fraction was employed, it is obvious that many different dose regimens can achieve a high tumor control rate and a satisfactory cosmesis. Periodically, systematic reviews appear in the literature giving readers good updates. Two more recent reviews at the time of writing of this chapter are a meta-analysis in *Radiotherapy and Oncology* [1] *and a systemic review in Dermatological Surgery* [2]. Here, we will examine two papers published decades apart to illustrate the different dose regimens historically used. They are chosen because of their large sample sizes and the widely separated time between their publications.

Fitzpatrick et al. published the experience at the Princess Margaret Hospital in 1984 of 1166 tumors of the eyelids treated "mostly" with superficial 100 kV X-rays [3]. About 90% were basal cell carcinomas (BCCs) and 10% squamous cell carcinomas (SCCs). Some tumors were treated with 125 kV, 250 kV, and up to Co-60 radiation, but the paper did not give a breakdown of numbers of patients treated with this more penetrating radiation. An approximate breakdown of the regimens used is listed in Table 4.1.

W. Kwan (✉)
Division of Radiation Oncology, Department of Surgery, Faculty of Medicine, University of British Columbia, Vancouver, BC, Canada
e-mail: wkwan@bccancer.bc.ca

K. J. Joseph et al. (eds.), *Radiotherapy in Skin Cancer*,
https://doi.org/10.1007/978-3-031-44316-9_4

Table 4.1 Dose fractionations used in external beam radiation treatment for skin cancers in the Fitzpatrick publication in 1984 [3]

Total dose (Gy)	Fractions	Days	Percent (number of patients/total)
20–22.5	1	1	25% (296/1166)
35–40	5	5–7	45% (524/1166)
42.5–45	10	12	22% (260/1166)
50–60	15–30	19–40	8% (86/1166)

Table 4.2 Longer dose fractionations used in the Marconi publication for skin cancer in 2016 [4]

Total dose (Gy)	Fractions	Percent (number of patients/total)
50	20	27% (273/1021)
55	20	18% (185/1021)
60	30	41% (419/1021)
Other	15–28	14% (144/1021)

Note that about 70% of patients received the course of radiation delivered in 1–5 fractions, and almost all patients were treated with superficial or orthovoltage X-rays (100 kV–250 kV). Protection of the eye was done in most patients by the insertion of a 2 mm lead shield into the conjunctival sac except for patients with very bulky tumors. The 5-year control rate was 95% for BCC and 93% for SCC. Cosmetic and functional results were "generally excellent" and "accepted by most patients." Overall complication rate was 9.6% with "fewer than half rated as serious." When the eye, particularly the anterior segment, was protected by shielding, ocular complications "did not follow."

More than three decades later, in 2016, Marconi et al. published their results on 1021 NMSCs (about 70% BCC, 30% SCC) treated with kilovoltage X-rays (80–200 kV) with longer fractionations [4] (Table 4.2). The tumors were from various head and neck locations with nose (34%), face (31%), eyelid/inner and outer canthi (21%), and pinna (7%) being the commonest sites. With a median follow-up of 44 months, the 5-year local control rates for BCC and SCC were 96% and 92%, respectively. The paper only reported on the acute toxicity of the treatment, which was 6% for RTOG Grade 3 or greater.

As illustrated in these two publications, both shorter and longer fractionations produce good results in treating NMSC. Most authors provide "expert opinions" on when to adopt which regimens:

1. Based on the volume of radiation: Field sizes up to 3–4 cm in largest dimension can be treated with 5 fractions or fewer, and up to 5–6 cm can be treated with 10 fractions, while for even larger field sizes or when it is necessary to include the deeper tissues and nodes, more standard 1.8–2.5 Gy fractions should ideally be used.
2. Based on the age of patients: Younger patients should be treated with more extended fractionations because of the concern of late soft tissue effects of larger dose per fractions. Depending on the availability of local surgical expertise,

some practitioners advocate a "no radiation, only surgery" approach in younger patients.

3. Based on the site: Certain sites are known to have a higher complication rate with radiotherapy such as anterior lower leg, dorsum of the hand, and, for some practitioners, pinna of the ear, where a lower dose per fraction may be recommended. (See more discussions under "f-factor for bone and cartilage" later in this chapter.) Some practitioners will elect not to treat the lower leg or dorsum of the hand with radiotherapy, whereas others will consider brachytherapy if treatment is required for the extremities [5].

A good review of the variation in the regimens used for radiotherapy of NMSC is a survey of the UK practice published in 2014 [6]. Eighteen dose fractionations were listed. The commonest are shown in Table 4.3, which can serve as an overall dose fractionation guide for everyday prescription.

Nonstandard Fractionations

While standard daily fractionations 5 days a week are most comfortable to practitioners, the patient population referred for radiotherapy for skin cancer tends to be older and often frail. It is not uncommon to see patients in their tenth decade of life with multiple comorbidities. As such, it is helpful to know the evidence supporting the use of less standard fractionations.

One Single Dose

Most radiation oncologists trained in the last 30 years are not used to delivering radiotherapy in one single treatment. However, the literature actually suggests that this is a safe and effective prescription. The Fitzpatrick series mentioned earlier in this chapter [3] reported on 296 patients treated with one single fraction of 20–22.5 Gy to a location surrounded by organs known to be sensitive to radiation (the eyelid). However, perhaps the most convincing evidence comes from the Nottingham series by Chan et al. [7]. This report described 1005 NMSCs treated with up to 10 years of follow-up. More than 97% of cancers were in the head and

Table 4.3 The most commonly used dose fractionations in radiotherapy of skin cancer in a large survey in the UK (McPartlin 2014) [5]. Please refer to the original publication for a complete list

Dose fractionation	Percentage of all responses
18–20 Gy/1 fraction	6%
35 Gy/5 fractions	25%
45 Gy/10 fractions	18%
55 Gy/20 fractions	14%

Adjuvant Dose Fractionation

Adjuvant radiotherapy is not infrequently prescribed after surgery for high-risk disease. Common indications include positive surgical margins, significant perineural invasion, bulky local disease (T3 or T4), and multiple nodal involvement. The reader is referred to a recent ASTRO guideline publication from 2020 [11] for a detailed discussion of various indications. The dose fractionation used in adjuvant therapy is dependent on the volume of tissue radiated. Thus, when a larger volume (for example, including the deep neck nodes for head and neck SCC) is radiated, protracted fractionations similar to the prevalent dose fractionation regimen for head and neck cancers are preferred. Common regimens include 60 Gy in 30 fractions for perceived higher residual tumor load and 50–52.5 Gy in 20 fractions for perceived lower microscopic residual tumor load. If a smaller volume is to be radiated, such as in the case of a positive surgical margin for primary disease, while standard 1.8–2 Gy fractions can be prescribed, hypofractionation such as 5 or 10 fractions can also be safely used. Some practitioners would reduce the curative dose by 10% for adjuvant treatment (e.g., 40 Gy in 10 fractions in the adjuvant setting rather than 45 Gy in 10 fractions in a curative setting).

Melanomas

Melanomas deserve special mention. Radiotherapy is rarely if ever used as curative treatment in a disease for which the standard of care is surgical excision. For selected very frail elderlies, primary radiotherapy has been used with success with lentigo maligna, a form of in situ melanoma typically affecting older individuals. A variety of dose/fractionation has been used in the literature, ranging from 35 Gy in 5 fractions to 50 Gy in 15 fractions if superficial X-rays were used [12]. While standard 1.8–2 Gy fractions can be used, lentigo maligna patients tend to be very old and may not tolerate a long course of radiotherapy. In addition, early radiobiological studies suggested a low α/β ratio for melanomas. Therefore, the author of this chapter favors the use of higher dose per fraction, similar to what is prescribed to NMSC of comparable sizes.

For invasive melanomas, radiotherapy is sometimes used after surgical nodal dissection if there is high-risk nodal involvement. Often, standard 1.8–2.0 Gy daily dose is prescribed to a total dose of 45–60 Gy depending on the perceived disease burden. The low α/β ratio for melanomas has led some institutions to use higher dose per fractions in adjuvant treatment. The MD Anderson has published their results a few times using a regimen of 30 Gy in 6 fractions delivered twice a week, as described by Guadagnolo et al. [13]. The good disease control and lack of toxicity make this a viable alternative dose fractionation to standard fractions.

References

1. Zaorsky NG, Lee CT, Zhang E, et al. Hypofractionated radiation therapy for basal and squamous cell skin cancer: a meta-analysis. Radiother Oncol. 2017;125:13–20.
2. Krausz A, Ji-Xu A, Smile T, et al. A systematic review of primary, adjuvant, and salvage radiation therapy for cutaneous squamous cell carcinoma. Dermatol Surg. 2021;47(5):587–92.
3. Fritzpatrick PJ, Thompson GA, Easterbrook WM, et al. Basal and squamous cell carcinoma of the eyelids and their treatment by radiotherapy. Int J Radiat Oncol Biol Phys. 1984;10(4):449–54.
4. Marconi DG, da Costa RB, Rauber E, et al. Head and neck non-melanoma skin cancer treated by superficial X-ray therapy: an analysis of 1021 cases. PLoS One. 2016;11(7):1–9. https://doi.org/10.1371/journal.pone.0156544.
5. Guinot JL, Rembielak A, Perez-Calatayud J, et al. GEC-ESTRO ACROP recommendations in skin brachytherapy. Radiother Oncol. 2018;126:377–85. https://doi.org/10.1016/j.radonc.2018.01.013.
6. McPartlin AJ, Slevin NF, Sykes AF, et al. Radiotherapy treatment of non-melanoma skin cancer: a survey of current UK practice and commentary. Br J Radiol. 2014;87:20140501. https://doi.org/10.1259/bjr.20140501.
7. Chan S, Dhadda AS, Swindell R. Single fraction radiotherapy for small superficial carcinoma of the skin. Clin Oncol. 2007;19:256–9.
8. Pampena R, Palmieri T, Kyrgidis A, et al. Orthovoltage radiotherapy for nonmelanoma skin cancer (NMSC): comparison between 2 different schedules. J Am Academy of Derm. 2016;74(2):341–7. https://doi.org/10.1016/j.jaad.2015.09.031.
9. Silva JJ, Tsang RW, Panzarella T, et al. Results of radiotherapy for epithelial skin cancer of the pinna: the Princess Margaret hospital experience, 1982–1993. Int J Radiat Oncol Biol Phys. 2000;47(2):451–9.
10. Hayter CRR, Lee KHY, Groome PA, et al. Necrosis following radiotherapy for carcinoma of the pinna. Int J Radiat Oncol Biol Phys. 1996;36(5):1033–7.
11. Likhjacheva A, Awan M, Barker CA, et al. Definitive and postoperative radiation therapy for basal and squamous cell cancers of the skin: executive summary of an American Society for Radiation Oncology clinical practice guideline. Pract Radiat Oncol. 2020;10:8–20.
12. Fogarty GB, Hong A, Scolyer RA, et al. Radiotherapy for lentigo maligna: a literature review and recommendations for treatment. Br J Dermatol. 2014;170(1):52–8. https://doi.org/10.1111/bjd.12611.
13. Guadagnolo BA, Prieto V, Weber R, et al. The role of adjuvant radiotherapy in the local management of desmoplastic melanoma. Cancer. 2014;120(9):1361–8.

Part II
Site-Specific Indications and Techniques

Chapter 5
Nasal Skin

Kurian Jones Joseph and Aswin George Abraham

Carcinoma of the skin of the nose accounts for about 25% of all carcinomas occurring in the head and neck region [1]. These cancers primarily arise from the nasal alae, the lateral surface, and the bridge of nose (Fig. 5.1). Basal cell carcinoma (BCC) is more common type followed by squamous cell carcinoma (SCC) (80% vs. 20% incidence, respectively).

Overall, 5% of patients with SCC develop lymph node metastasis, and the incidence according to stage is as follows: 3% for T1, 6% for T2, and 13% for T3 or higher stage [2]. Typically, nodal metastases are not seen from BCC.

Primary radiotherapy and surgery are the treatment options for carcinoma of nasal skin that provide comparable results for early-stage disease (T1 and T2). Cure with preservation of function and cosmesis are the fundamental considerations in treatment decision. Because these cancers have a high chance of cure with various treatments, cosmetic outcome is the priority.

Primary radiotherapy preserves nasal anatomy and is preferred over surgery since the nasal skin is closely adherent to the underlying cartilage with poor elasticity and could affect cosmetic outcomes following surgery. Nasal cartilage is considered fairly resistant to radiation [3]. However, use of inappropriate radiation technique and dose fractionation could result in undesirable treatment-related sequelae.

K. J. Joseph (✉)
Department of Oncology, University of Alberta, Edmonton, Canada

Division of Radiation Oncology, Cross Cancer Institute, Edmonton, Canada
e-mail: kurian.joseph@albertahealthservices.ca

A. G. Abraham
Division of Radiation Oncology, Cross Cancer Institute, Edmonton, Canada
e-mail: aswin.abraham@albertahealthservices.ca

K. J. Joseph et al. (eds.), *Radiotherapy in Skin Cancer*,
https://doi.org/10.1007/978-3-031-44316-9_5

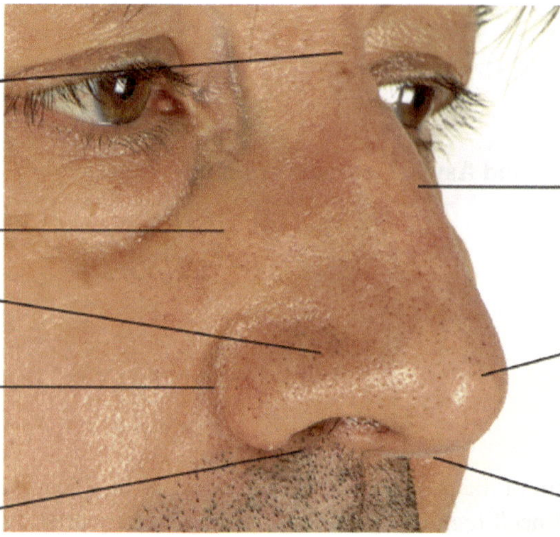

Fig. 5.1 Distribution of tumors of nasal skin (Modified from Mazeron et al., with permission)

Indications for Radiotherapy

Primary radiotherapy is offered for all stages of carcinoma of the nose, particularly in elderly patients who may not be suitable for radical surgery due to medical comorbidities.

Adjuvant radiotherapy is offered postoperatively when patient presents with:

T3/T4 disease
Residual disease after surgery
Positive margin (margins ≥2 mm are considered adequate)
Perineural or lymphovascular invasion
Involvement of regional lymph nodes
Patients with two or more risk factors including tumor >2 cm, poor differentiation, depth/thickness ≥4 mm, desmoplastic or infiltrative growth pattern with immunosuppression

Treatment Approach

T1 and T2 BCC and SCC are curable with primary radiotherapy. The selection of the appropriate radiotherapy modality is influenced by a number of factors such as tumor site, size and depth of the lesion, previous surgery, institutional availability, expertise, and patient convenience. The orthovoltage radiotherapy is the commonly used radiotherapy modality that allows full dose of radiation over the skin surface. Electron irradiation is not commonly used because of the small field size, skin-sparing effect, irregularity of the skin surface, and heterogeneity of the tissues within the treatment field (skin vs. cartilage vs. bone and air).

Brachytherapy (refer to the brachytherapy section) and orthovoltage radiotherapy produce similar outcomes for T1 tumors and are used in routine clinical practice. Brachytherapy delivers a higher tumor dose resulting in better local control over a shorter treatment time [4]. For T2 tumor, orthovoltage irradiation is usually more suitable. For tumors larger than 4 cm, megavoltage irradiation is preferred, while brachytherapy or orthovoltage irradiation could be reserved for a boost dose.

The irregularity of the skin surface and the heterogeneity of the tissues (skin vs. cartilage vs. bone) make brachytherapy the technique of choice for vestibular tumors. For tumors over the lateral surface, orthovoltage radiotherapy is preferred.

Treatment Planning

Target Volume

The target volume encompasses the primary tumor with an adequate margin of 1–1.5 cm. Lymph node metastases are uncommon, and hence lymph node regions are not electively included in the target volume after adequate staging. For T3 or higher tumors, CT or PET/CT imaging or sentinel lymph node biopsy is suggested in the literature to evaluate nodal status. Node-negative patient will be offered close surveillance, whereas radical neck dissection is offered for node-positive cases. Generally, adjuvant radiotherapy will be offered for this group of patients (refer Chap. 14 for details).

During treatment planning, special note should be made of the fact that deeper infiltration of tumor can occur at the region of embryonic fusion planes, which include inner canthus, nasolabial fold, and philtrum. Hence, adequate margin should be given to the target volume to avoid geographical miss for tumors in these regions.

Clinical markup is done to define target volume, which is usually 1–1.5 cm margin around the primary tumor, which accommodates for regions at risk and day-to-day setup variation (Fig. 5.2).

Treatment setup and field arrangement:

Generally, treatment is delivered by orthovoltage technique. Patients are positioned supine, in a comfortable position, and a single direct radiation field is used for treatment delivery. The dose is prescribed at the skin surface, and the target should be covered by at least 90% isodose line. External eye shield or nostril shields are used to minimize dose to septum and nasal floor. Shielding is also used to protect the upper gum if indicated.

If the patient is treated with high-energy photons or electron treatment, CT-based planning is recommended. The patient must be immobilized lying supine in a custom shell, and 3 mm CT slices should be acquired from the top of the orbit to the level of hyoid bone. The lesion should be marked by a lead wire before CT scanning

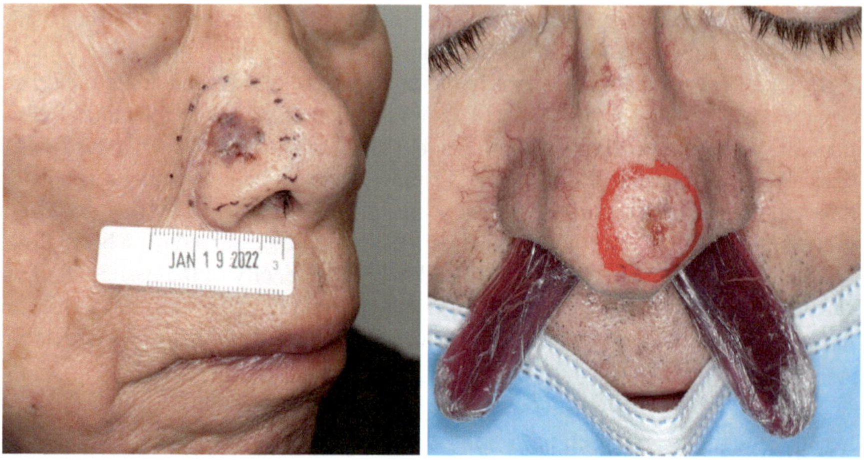

Fig. 5.2 Orthovoltage radiotherapy delivered through a direct field. Lead shield is used to protect the nasal floor in figure on the right side

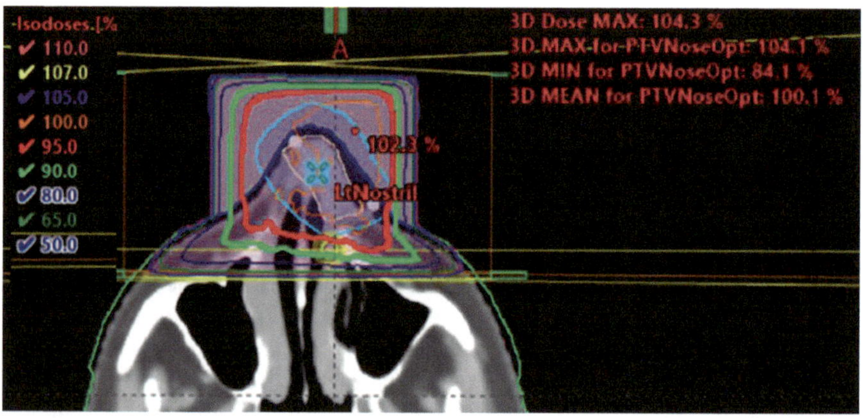

Fig. 5.3 Beam arrangement for tumor involving both sides (mainly over the left) of the bridge of nose. Wax block is used for homogenous dose distribution

to visualize the lesion in the planning scan. The clinical target volume (CTV) is defined by adding an isotropic 10 mm margin around the gross tumor volume (GTV) while editing to avoid expansion beyond natural tumor barriers and air cavity. A PTV margin of 2–5 mm is added around CTV for day-to-day setup variation.

Typically, 3-dimensional conformal radiotherapy (3D-CRT) using lateral opposed photon beam arrangement is used to treat lesion involving both sides of the nose (Fig. 5.3). Wax bolus is used on the surface of nasal skin (and upper lip) to produce homogenous dose distribution.

Traditional radiotherapy techniques do not spare the nasal septum, which is a dose-limiting structure. Volumetric modulated arc therapy (VMAT) can be used to limit dose to nasal septum and minimize skin toxicity, especially when the target is the whole nose (Fig. 5.4).

A single direct field can be used for electron radiotherapy. For electrons, a bolus is used over the skin surface to achieve adequate surface dose, and the target volume will be covered at the minimum, by 90% isodose line.

Brachytherapy (refer to the brachytherapy section).

Dose

The dose and treatment scheme are discussed in the general sections (Chap. 5).

Hypofractionated dose schedules are commonly used and are well tolerated. Moderate hypofractionation (dose 2.5–3 Gy/fraction) is recommended for younger patients. The NCCN (Version 1.2022) recommendations are:

T1 tumor: 50–55 Gy/15–20 fractions/3–4 weeks
T2, T3, T4/with invasion of bone or deep tissue: 45–55 Gy/15–20 fractions/3–4 weeks; 60–70 Gy/30–35 fractions/6–7 weeks
Adjuvant RT: 60–64 Gy/30–32 fractions/6–7 weeks; 50 Gy/20 Fractions/4 Weeks
Other commonly used regimens are: 4000–4500/10 fractions; 3000–3500/5/1 weeks

Higher dose fractions over 4–6 Gy and short treatment time (≤5 days) are associated with risk of cartilage necrosis [5].

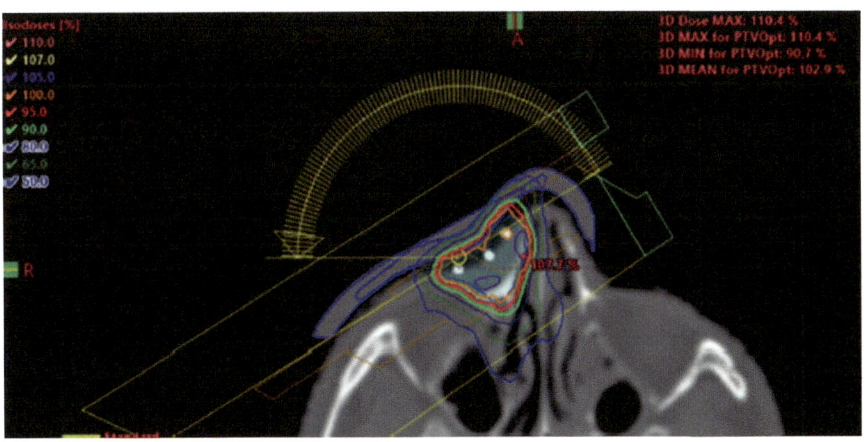

Fig. 5.4 VMAT plan for a large linear lesion on the right side of the nose. Bolus used to achieve adequate skin dose

Treatment-related Side Effects

Nasal functions are affected by radiation, and the common acute side effects following radiotherapy are:

- Soreness of the nasal cavity
- Nose bleeding and crusting
- Dry nose
- Dysosmia or dysgeusia

These symptoms are temporary, and various medications used to treat acute symptoms include:

- Topical 0.5–1% steroid cream
- Saline or steroid nasal spray
- Analgesics

Skin necrosis is more frequent following brachytherapy, and the incidence is <5%. Commonly occurring late treatment-related side effects are:

- Skin pallor
- Skin atrophy
- Dyschromia
- Telangiectasia

These side effects are progressive with time and generally asymptomatic [6]. High risk of osteoradionecrosis and radiochondritis with orthovoltage RT has been reported in the past. However, various experts indicated that the nasal cartilage has a high radiation tolerance, and the risk is very small when using properly fractionated schedules.

Outcomes

Primary radiotherapy resulted in 93–95% local control with satisfactory cosmesis [1].

The predictors for local control are tumor size (T = <2 cm vs. >2–4 cm vs. >4 cm), tumor site (lateral surface, 94% vs. vestibule, 88%), and histology (BCC vs. SCC).

References

1. Caccialanza M, Piccinno R, Percivalle S, Rozza M. Radiotherapy of carcinomas of the skin overlying the cartilage of the nose: our experience in 671 lesions. J Eur Acad Dermatol Venereol. 2009;23:1044–9.

2. Mazeron JJ, Chassagne D, Crook J, et al. Radiation therapy of carcinomas of the skin of nose and nasal vestibule: a report of 1676 cases by the Groupe Europeen de Curiethérapie. Radiother Oncol. 1988;13:165–73.
3. Bussu F, Tagliaferri L, Piras A, et al. Multidisciplinary approach to nose vestibule malignancies: setting new standards. Acta Otorhinolaryngol Ital. 2021;41:S158–65.
4. Czerwinski MD, Jansen PP, Zwijnenburg EM, et al. Radiotherapy as nose preservation treatment strategy for cancer of the nasal vestibule: the Dutch experience. Radiother Oncol. 2021;164:20–6.
5. Hayter CR, Lee KH, Groome PA, Brundage MD. Necrosis following radiotherapy for carcinoma of the pinna. Int J Radiat Oncol Biol Phys. 1996;36:1033–7.
6. Tsao MN, Tsang RW, Liu FF, Panzarella T, Rotstein L. Radiotherapy management for squamous cell carcinoma of the nasal skin: the Princess Margaret Hospital experience. Int J Radiat Oncol Biol Phys. 2002;52:973–9.

Chapter 6
Scalp

M. J. Veness

Introduction

Non-melanoma skin cancer (NMSC) comprises predominantly basal cell carcinoma (BCC) and cutaneous squamous cell carcinoma (cSCC) and is the most common malignancy worldwide. The sun-exposed scalp is a site where cSCC arises more often than BCC, with most patients being older males, many with an extensive history of NMSC. In female patients, scalp NMSC is more often BCC. Patients with operable lesions should be recommended surgery; there is a subset of patients with cSCC at risk of developing local recurrence that may benefit from adjuvant radiotherapy (RT) [1, 2]. Patients not considered surgical candidates should be considered for RT alone and potentially be cured, even in the setting of an advanced primary care centre [3, 4].

Managing patients with cSCC of the scalp poses site-specific issues in terms of anatomical restrictions limiting deep resection and often large areas requiring treatment and associated contour changes (Fig. 6.1). The relatively thin soft tissue structures have implications for obtaining a negative deep excision margin, which may necessitate removal of the periosteum or outer table of the skull with transposition flap reconstruction. Extension into the cranial cavity at diagnosis (stage T4 lesion) is uncommon but documented and may require neurosurgical intervention if suitable [4].

The relevance of margin status in cSCC in terms of both treatment and outcome remains unclear with limited high-level evidence. Margin status (clear vs. positive) has been shown to have an impact on recurrence and outcome, with incomplete

M. J. Veness (✉)
Department of Radiation Oncology, Crown Princess Mary Cancer Centre, Westmead Hospital, Sydney, NSW, Australia

University of Sydney, Sydney, NSW, Australia
e-mail: michael.veness@health.nsw.gov.au

K. J. Joseph et al. (eds.), *Radiotherapy in Skin Cancer*,
https://doi.org/10.1007/978-3-031-44316-9_6

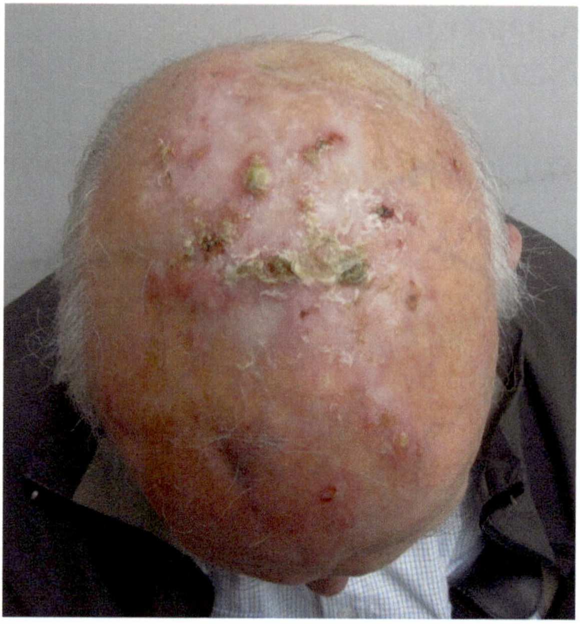

Fig. 6.1 Typical appearance of an older male with a chronically sun-damaged scalp exhibiting large areas of actinic changes likely to also involve in situ and invasive cSCC. Patients nearly always have undergone multiple previous treatment that may have included RT

excision proposed as an additional high-risk feature for poor outcome in high-risk patients [2].

The scalp is a site where skin field cancerisation (SFC) occurs, a not well-defined entity, which includes wide areas of chronically ultraviolet-damaged skin exhibiting a spectrum of changes that may include multiple actinic keratosis, in situ cSCC and invasive cSCC [5] (see also Fig. 6.1). Whole or partial scalp RT for SFC, which can be safely delivered utilising modern highly conformal RT, has been proposed by some as an option in select patients, but remains controversial [6].

Indications for Radiotherapy

Radiotherapy is an effective adjuvant modality in patients with NMSC at risk of developing local recurrence and a definitive/palliative option in patients who are not candidates for scalp surgery (or more extensive re-excision surgery).

A clear role and benefit of adjuvant RT for improving local control and possibly survival in the setting of close or involved margins in cSCC are contentious but should be considered. Patients considered at risk of developing local recurrence often have multiple unfavourable pathological features but with an involved/close margin often being the most relevant factor [7].

Adjuvant

Pathological risk factors for locoregional recurrence include margin status, tumour thickness, invasion beyond subcutaneous fat, presence of perineural invasion (PNI), diameter >20 mm, and poor differentiation in addition to immunosuppression and recurrent setting [8]. Unlike BCC where a patient with a close or involved margin is at risk of local relapse only and observation with expectant treatment (i.e. RT or surgery) is an accepted option in many, further treatment is generally recommended for an involved or close cSCC margin due to the increased risk of developing local recurrence, which in turn increases the risk of subsequent nodal metastases [9] (Fig. 6.2). The definition of a close excision margin prompting further treatment is unclear, and patients will often have multiple unfavourable features present.

Definitive

Patients considered medically or technically inoperable may still be considered for radical intent RT. The scalp is not a functional unit similar to the lip or eyelids, but patients may decline surgery if reconstruction is required. Patients with extensive lesions, even involving bone invasion, are potentially curable with RT alone.

Palliative

Elderly unwell patients with locally advanced symptomatic (bleeding, painful) lesions will benefit from RT with the aim to improve their quality of life by obtaining growth restraint and a durable reduction in the treated cSCC. A

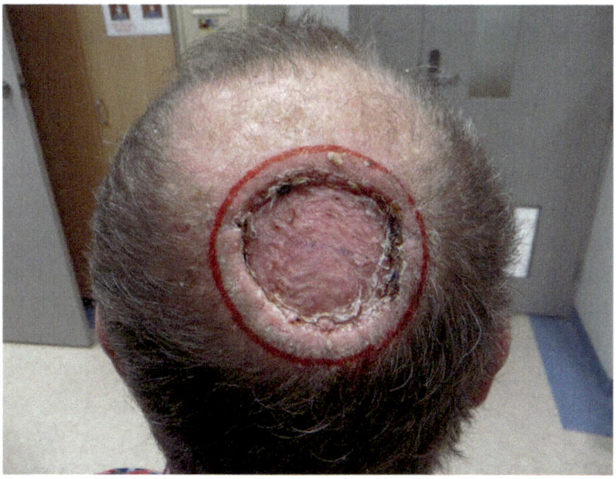

Fig. 6.2 73-Year-old male post-wide local excision of a 25 mm moderately differentiated cSCC with a close 0.2 mm deep margin and PNI present beyond the actual lesion. A recommendation of adjuvant RT was made, and he received 50 Gy in 20 fractions using superficial energy photons (125 kVp) with a 1 cm field margin placed beyond the graft site

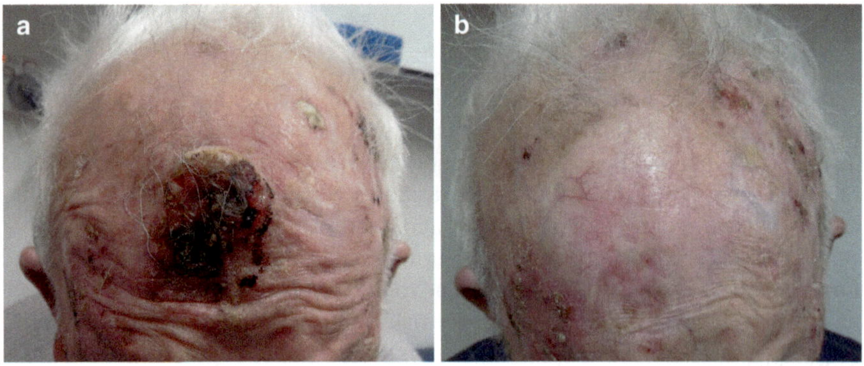

Fig. 6.3 (**a**) 85-Year-old male of poor performance status with a large poorly mobile anterior scalp cSCC. He was deemed medically inoperable and proceeded to RT alone receiving 36 Gy in 6 fractions delivered twice per week using orthovoltage energy photons (300 kVp) and a 2 cm field margin. (**b**) 3 months post-RT, the patient has experienced complete clinical regression. Note the in-field hypopigmentation, scattered telangiectasia and epidermal atrophy

hypofractionated approach of 5–6 fractions is well tolerated and effective in achieving an excellent response (Fig. 6.3a, b).

Treatment Approach

The optimal RT treatment modality for scalp cSCC is dependent on lesion size/thickness and location. Relatively small fields (2–5 cm circle) on flat surfaces (e.g. lateral scalp, vertex) may be treated with superficial/orthovoltage energy photons (125–300 kVp) or alternatively low/moderate-energy electrons (6–9 MeV) (4–6 cm circle) with the addition of tissue equivalent bolus (0.5–1 cm). The aim is for the prescribed dose to be delivered down to the level of the periosteum. Patients with skin grafts may only require superficial energy photons or low-energy electrons, while those with flap reconstruction usually require moderate-energy electrons or megavoltage photons (see below).

Three-dimensional megavoltage conformal RT (3D-CRT), highly conformal intensity-modulated RT (IMRT) or volumetric arc therapy (VMAT) is often the optimal approach and allows for the treatment of extensive areas of scalp (including whole scalp), if warranted (Fig. 6.4a–c). By using modern RT techniques, the dose delivered to underlying structures within the cranial cavity can be accurately measured with the aim to minimise the dose received. The curvature of the scalp often limits the use of large electron fields but not IMRT/VMAT. Similar to using electrons, tissue equivalent bolus is required to increase the skin dose and may involve the use of 3D printed bolus [10].

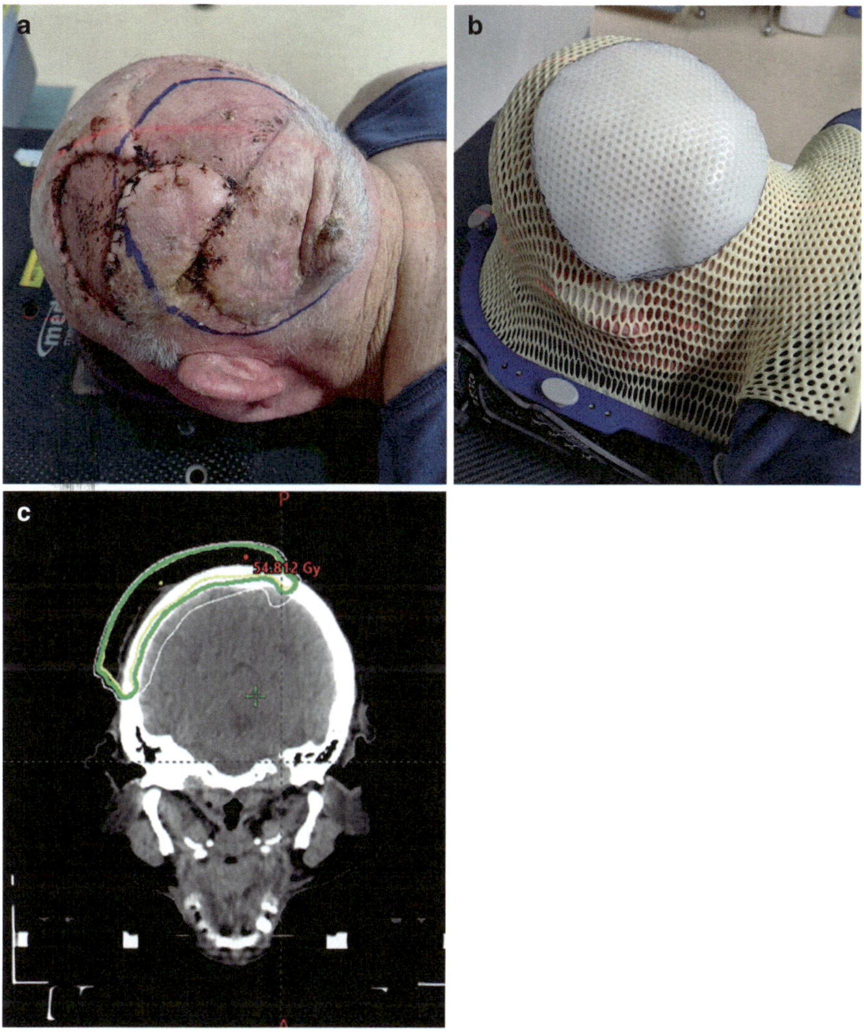

Fig. 6.4 (**a**) 67-Year-old male post-op after extensive posterior scalp surgery in the setting of a large recurrent cSCC with multiple deep involved margins. Note the rotation scalp flap as part of his reconstruction. The patient was prescribed 50 Gy in 20 fractions using a VMAT RT approach. The solid blue line delineates where 1 cm of tissue equivalent bolus will be placed. (**b**) Patient in Fig. 6.4a is positioned prone and immobilised in a thermoplastic mask with bolus placed directly onto the mask prior to CT simulation. (**c**) Isodose plan for patient in Fig. 6.4a, b with the green isodose illustrating 95% isodose distribution highlighting the precise delivery of the prescribed dose of RT. Note the ability to achieve a uniform distribution despite the curvature of the scalp and underlying skull

Treatment Planning

Target Volume

Local Treatment

It is important that the prescribed dose is delivered to the skin surface as well as at depth. Bolus (0.5–1 cm) is required if using megavoltage photons or electrons. Accepting anatomical barriers, such as bone, patients should be treated with at least 2 cm margins especially peripherally beyond a lesion (GTV) or surgical bed to achieve a clinical target volume (CTV). In the presence of extensive PNI, wider margins (3–4 cm) may be required but, unlike in other sites of the head and neck, may not involve treating named neural pathways or skull base. The exception is supra-orbital cSCC with PNI. The CTV can be cropped at anatomical barriers to limit dose to critical structures such as the brain. CTV at depth should be down to the periosteum or skull outer table, unless involved. Planning target volume (PTV) expansions of 3–5 mm are recommended. If clinicians utilise electrons, wider field margins (2–3 cm) are required and dose is prescribed to 90% isodose line.

Palliative

The aim of palliative radiotherapy is to treat the GTV with adequate but limited field margins of usually 1–2 cm. Lesions may be advanced and deeply invasive and require the use of megavoltage photons or electrons.

Dose

The dose fractionation schedules prescribed are similar whether the setting is adjuvant or definitive. Hypofractionation similarly remains an option in both settings, especially in older poor performance patients. Ideally, adjuvant RT should commence in 4–6 weeks following surgery, and skin grafts should be completely healed to reduce the risk of graft loss.

Adjuvant

The role of hypofractionation has been well proven in treating NMSC, and doses of 45–50 Gy in 2.5–3 Gy fractions are recommended in the adjuvant setting. If using 2 Gy fractions, a total dose of 56–60 Gy is recommended. Short-course hypofractionation in the adjuvant setting is an option in elderly patients with high-risk lesions.

Definitive

Patients considered inoperable may still be considered for radical intent RT. Those of good performance status should be offered treatment involving an extended 5–6-week course of RT (e.g. 55–60 Gy in 2–2.2 Gy fractions). Older good performance patients can still be recommended radical intent RT that may involve 3–4 weeks of moderate hypofractionation (e.g. 45–50 Gy in 2.5–3 Gy fractions) [11].

Palliative

In elderly patients, short-course hypofractionated RT confers no disadvantage in regard to outcome when compared to more protracted schedules. In most patients, 5–7 Gy fractions delivered 1–3 fractions per week to a total dose of 30–40 Gy result in excellent local control rates and very tolerable toxicity [12, 13]. Other hypofractionated regimes, involving 1–3 larger (8–10 Gy) fractions delivered once per week, can also be considered efficacious in poor performance patients.

Treatment-Related Side Effects

In-field moist desquamation is typical for any patient receiving a radical dose of RT. Acute reactions tend to peak shortly after completion of RT and last for 2–3 weeks. Topical emollients such as Sorbolene are recommended during treatment, and topical burn-type dressings should be used in the setting of moist desquamation. In-field alopecia, hypopigmentation, epidermal atrophy and telangiectasia are all likely to arise following high-dose RT. The late in-field development of osteoradionecrosis secondary to skin graft loss occurs in a minority and is unpredictable and although associated with bone exposure is often asymptomatic (Fig. 6.5). Patients developing osteoradionecrosis are often smokers and diabetics and may have a history of vascular disease.

Outcomes

There are limited outcome data specific to patients with scalp cSCC; however, the Peter MacCallum Cancer Centre, Melbourne, reported on the outcome of 233 scalp cSCC patients treated with either surgery (45%), RT (26%) or both (26%) and documented a 5-year disease-specific and progression-free survival of 94% and 51%, respectively [14]. The 5-year cumulative incidence of local and regional relapse was 11% and 7%, respectively, and noting only four patients eventually developed distant metastases.

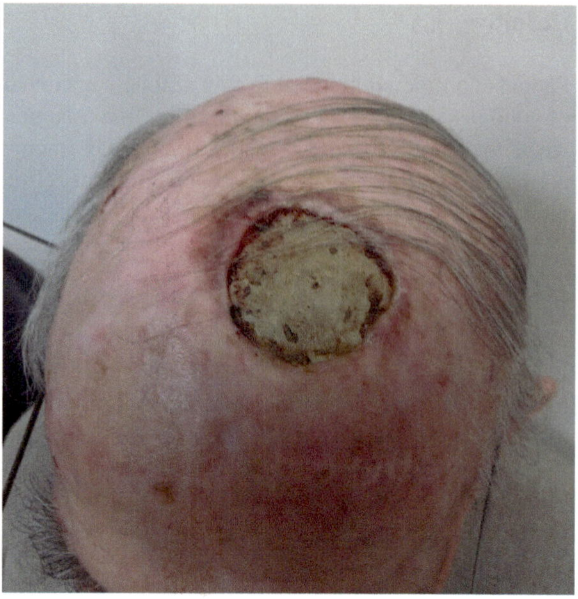

Fig. 6.5 Skull exposure following excision and adjuvant radiotherapy for a cSCC with an involved deep margin. The exposed area reflects complete loss of a skin graft and also delineates the radiotherapy field. Note the well-defined border that defines the previous RT field. The patient was asymptomatic and declined any intervention

Follow-Up

Patients should be clinically reviewed 3–4 monthly for the first 2 years and 6 monthly thereafter for 2–3 years. Those undergoing extensive surgery involving flap reconstruction may benefit from cross-sectional imaging as deep flap recurrence may not be asymptomatic until advanced.

References

1. Veness MJ, Delishaj D, Barnes EA, Bezugly A, Rembielak A. Current role of radiotherapy in non-melanoma skin cancer. Clin Oncol. 2019;31:749–58.
2. Mendis RL, Morgan G, Abdul-Razak M, Wong E, Howle J, Gebski V, Veness M. Margin status predicts outcome in patients with cutaneous squamous cell carcinoma of the scalp: the Westmead hospital experience. Skin. 2022;6:295–302.
3. Xing D, Hettige S, Chee LYS, Nair R, Hegde R. Curative radiotherapy for locally advanced scalp squamous cell carcinoma. Cureus. 2021;13(10):e18514.
4. Gruber I, Koelbl O. Dramatic radiotherapy response of a giant T4 cutaneous squamous cell carcinoma of the scalp with extensive bone destruction: a case report. J Med Case Rep. 2021;15:610. https://doi.org/10.1186/s13256-021-03213-6.
5. Daly T, Veness M, Poulsen M, Muir J, De'Ambrosis B, Kennedy D. Wide-field radiation therapy for skin cancerisation—have we forgotten what we learned? JMIRO. 2022;67:128.
6. Fogarty GB, Young S, Lo S, et al. Field-based radiotherapy using volumetric modulated arc therapy (VMAT) for skin field cancerisation (SFC)-outcomes from 100 fields. Int J Radiol Radiat Ther. 2021;8:13–24.

7. Petre A, Pommier P, Brahmi T, Chabaud S, et al. Benefit from adjuvant radiotherapy according to the number of risk factors in cutaneous squamous cell carcinoma. Radio Oncol. 2022;168:53–60.
8. Zhang J, Wang Y, Wijaya Z, Chen J. Efficacy and prognostic factors of adjuvant radiotherapy for cutaneous squamous cell carcinoma: a systemic review and meta-analysis. J Eur Acad Dermatol Venerol. 2021;35:1777–87.
9. Howle JR, Morgan GJ, Kalnins I, Palme CE, Veness MJ. Metastatic cutaneous squamous cell carcinoma of the scalp. ANZ J Surg. 2008;78:449–53.
10. Hsu EJ, Parsons D, Chiu T, Godley AR, Sher DJ, Vo DT. 3D printed integrated bolus/headrest for radiation therapy for malignancies involving the posterior scalp and neck. 3D Print Med. 2022;8:22.
11. Tsao MN, Barnes EA, Karam I, Rembielak A. Hypofractionated radiation therapy in keratinocyte carcinoma. Clin Oncol. 2022;34:e218–24.
12. De Felice F, Musio D, De Falco D, et al. Definitive weekly hypofractionated radiotherapy in cutaneous squamous cell carcinoma: response rates and outcomes in elderly patients unfit for surgery. Int J Dermatol. 2022;61:911–5.
13. Veness M. Hypofractionated radiotherapy in older patients with non-melanoma skin cancer: less is better. Australas J Dermatol. 2018;59:124–7.
14. Estall V, Allen A, Webb A, Bressel M, McCormack C, Spillane J. Outcomes following management of squamous cell carcinoma of the scalp: a retrospective series of 235 patients treated at the Peter MacCallum Cancer Centre. Australas J Dermatol. 2017;58:e207–15.

Chapter 7
Eyelid

Gerald B. Fogarty

Adequate eyelid function is essential for effective vision. The eyelid is mainly skin and glandular tissue. The eyelid is an RT target when tumours arising from the tissues of the eyelid require RT treatment. The usual cancers are therefore skin cancers and adenocarcinoma, especially sebaceous gland adenocarcinoma (SGC). In terms of the types of cancer encountered, a retrospective study investigating the clinicopathological analysis of 5146 eyelid tumours found, of 768 malignant tumours, 49% basal cell carcinoma (BCC), 34% sebaceous gland carcinoma (SGC), 12% squamous cell carcinoma (SCC), 3% malignant melanoma (MM), and 1% lymphoma [1].

RT is often used as a definitive or an adjuvant treatment to achieve tissue conservation and to achieve with adequate function and cosmesis. Multidisciplinary care involving pre-RT assessment and follow-up by an ophthalmologist is suggested when RT is contemplated.

Anatomy and Histology of the Eyelid as Relevant to RT

The eyelids are thin folds of skin that cover the eyes. The superior eyelid extends to the eyebrow, and the inferior lid extends below the inferior orbital rim to join the cheek. The eyelids are separated by the palpebral fissure and meet at the medial and lateral canthi. The levator palpebrae superioris muscle retracts the superior eyelid. The eyelid external surface is skin, and this features a row of eyelashes along the eyelid margins. The internal surfaces are the conjunctiva.

G. B. Fogarty (✉)
The Icon Cancer Centre, Sydney, NSW, Australia

University of Technology, Sydney, NSW, Australia
e-mail: Gerald.Fogarty@icon.team

K. J. Joseph et al. (eds.), *Radiotherapy in Skin Cancer*,
https://doi.org/10.1007/978-3-031-44316-9_7

Important anatomical relationships include the lacrimal glands supero-laterally in the orbit, supplying reflexive tears. Immediately posterior to the eyelids are the anterior chambers of the eye including the cornea, iris, ciliary body, and lens. When the eye is in a neutral position, these structures are central while the surrounding sclera is peripheral. The anterior chamber can be moved voluntarily by cooperative patients medially, laterally, superiorly, and inferiorly to a peripheral position by the extraocular muscles for the duration of an external beam fraction. Figure 7.1 illustrates sagittal section through the anterior orbit showing the cross-sectional anatomy of the eyelids.

Histologically, the eyelids comprise, from superficial to deep, keratinizing skin which is usually only 1 mm thick, subcutaneous tissue, orbicularis oculi muscle, orbital septum and tarsal plates, a mucous membrane that is a continuation of the keratinizing squamous epithelium of the outside skin, and, lastly, palpebral conjunctiva. This hugs the inside of the eyelid, reflecting on itself to form the bulbar conjunctiva that covers the anterior sclera except for the cornea. The conjunctiva is composed of non-keratinized, stratified squamous epithelium. The meibomian or tarsal glands lie within the tarsal plates and secrete the lipid part of the tear film that channels tears into the naso-lacrimal duct. Primary cancers can arise from all these layers.

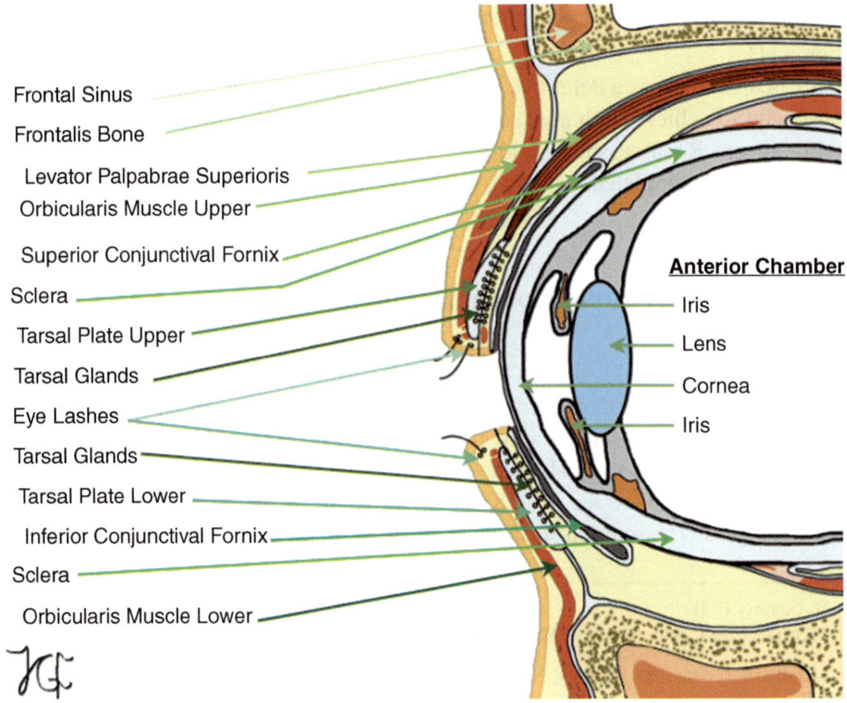

Fig. 7.1 Sagittal section through the anterior orbit showing the cross-sectional anatomy of the eyelid

Knowledge of the lymph drainage and nerve supply is important in defining RT treatment volumes and in knowing what and where to assess for recurrence during post-RT follow-up appointments. The lymph drainage from the medial end of both eyelids is towards the submandibular nodes, and the lateral ends towards the pre-auricular nodes. See Fig. 7.2. Tumours can spread by perineural invasion, so knowledge of the innervation of the eyelid is needed for RT volume delineation. Nerve supply is via three cranial nerves (III, V, VII) and sympathetic nerve fibres. Sensory fibres for the superior eyelid enter the skull through the supraorbital foramen, the opening of which can be palpated along the medial superior rim of the orbit. This foramen can be filled when a superior eyelid tumour is locally advanced by perineural invasion. The supraorbital nerve runs superiorly along the medial side of the orbit above the levator palpebrae superioris and can be expanded on MRI when involved with tumour, which is often associated with paraesthesia and formication of the medial forehead. Sensory fibres for the inferior eyelid enter the skull via the inferior orbital nerve as it enters the infraorbital canal of the maxilla and runs along the floor of the orbit. Perineural symptoms of paraesthesia and formication need to be asked about at presentation and follow-up.

Physiologically, the eyelids spread the tears and other secretions on the eye surface to keep it moist on blinking. Resting moisture comes from glands on and in the eyelid, and reactive moisture or reflexive tears come from the lacrimal glands. The meibomian glands secrete a lipid-rich fluid which guides tears. This and the adherence of the cornea to the lower lid are essential to drain the tears towards the

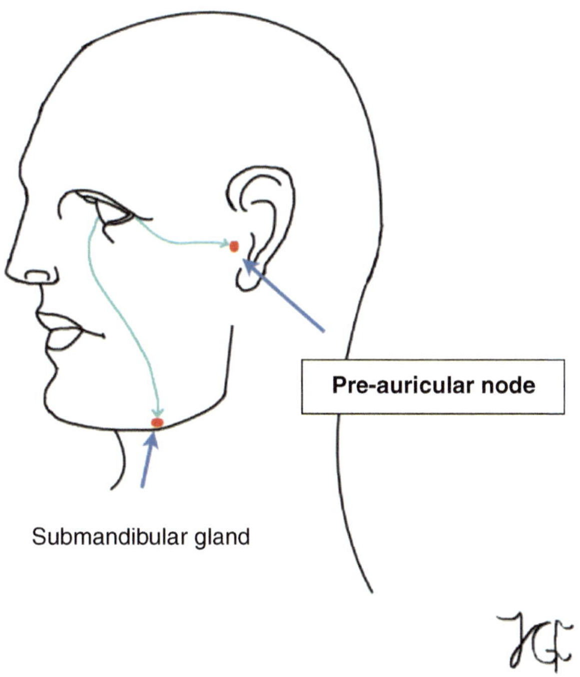

Fig. 7.2 The lymph drainage from the medial end of both eyelids is towards the submandibular nodes, and the lateral ends towards the pre-auricular nodes

lacrimal papillae and then into the nose via the naso-lacrimal duct. At the medial end of both eyelids are small rises called the lacrimal papillae through which lacrimal fluid exits into the naso-lacrimal ducts that terminate in the inferior turbinates of the nose. The lids with their eyelashes protect the bulb, especially through the blink reflex. Common pathological terms applied to the eyelids include entropion, which is a turning in of the lid so that eyelash hairs can irritate the eye. Ectropion is a turning out of the lid associated with tears falling over the edge of the lower lid, a process called epiphora. This happens especially when the lid is not abutting the cornea. Blepharospasm is a twitching eyelid.

Indications for Radiotherapy and Treatment Approach

The indications and oncological outcomes for RT to the eyelid are similar to those outlined in the chapter "Nasal Skin" in this book. Definitive RT to conventionally fractionated 60 Gy is often attempted for the more radiation-sensitive tumours of BCC and cSCC to achieve acceptable tissue conservation, function, and cosmesis. This is based on retrospective studies such as Petsuksiri et al. [2] who treated SCC of the eyelid with curative intent RT, 32 definitively and 10 with adjuvant post-operative RT (PORT). Surviving patients were followed for a median of 76 months. At 5 years, local, regional, and distant disease control rates for all tumours were 88%, 95%, and 97%, respectively. There was no difference in outcome between definitive and PORT cases. Definitive RT may be attempted for eyelid melanoma in situ (MIS) when tissue sacrifice is not wanted or possible [3].

PORT is recommended for the more radiation-resistant tumours such as SGC and malignant melanoma. Takagawa et al. [4], in a retrospective study of 83 patients with eyelid SGC, treated 65 (78%) with definitive RT and 18 with PORT for recurrence or positive surgical margins, all to a median dose of 60 Gy. At a median follow-up of 92.1 months, 36 patients (43.3%) developed local recurrence. The 7-year overall survival, freedom from neck lymph node recurrence, and local control rates were 83.5%, 75.5%, and 52.3%, respectively. Tumour size ≤10 mm achieved superior outcomes with definitive RT, and with larger lesions treated with PORT. Hata et al. [5], in 13 patients with eyelid SGC treated with definitive intent RT to a median dose of 60 Gy, achieved in-field local control of all tumours at a median follow-up period of 55 months.

Treatment Planning

The target volume depends on tumour location and, for definitive RT, GTV plus 0.5 cm expansion to CTV. The CTV for PORT is 1 cm around the eyelid scar. PTV expansion is modality dependent in both scenarios. Superficial RT (SXRT) expansion to field is typically 5–10 mm and for electrons is 1–1.5 cm. Expansions may be less due to a desire to limit the conjunctival volume being irradiated to decrease the risk of xerophthalmia. Megavoltage photon RT is not commonly used but does play a selective role. See Fig. 7.3.

Traditionally, the eyelid has been treated with an internal eye shield in place to protect the anterior structures of the eye. See Fig. 7.4. This involves putting local anaesthetic drops in the eye followed by insertion of the shield. The best way to insert the shield is to ask the patient to look medially and then carefully slip the superior part of the shield as laterally as possible and as far as possible under the superior lid, and then insert the inferior part of the shield under the lower lid and then ask the patient to relax. The shield settles in the middle of the eye. A lead shield covered in acrylic coating is used for SXRT, and a tungsten shield similarly coated is used for electrons. Electron energies 9 MeV or less are used to avoid unnecessary penetration and penumbra, but they do require bolus to achieve surface dose to the lid, making it a complicated procedure. Recently, a technique was developed to treat eyelid cancer with RT in cooperative patients, without the use of an internal eye shield [6].

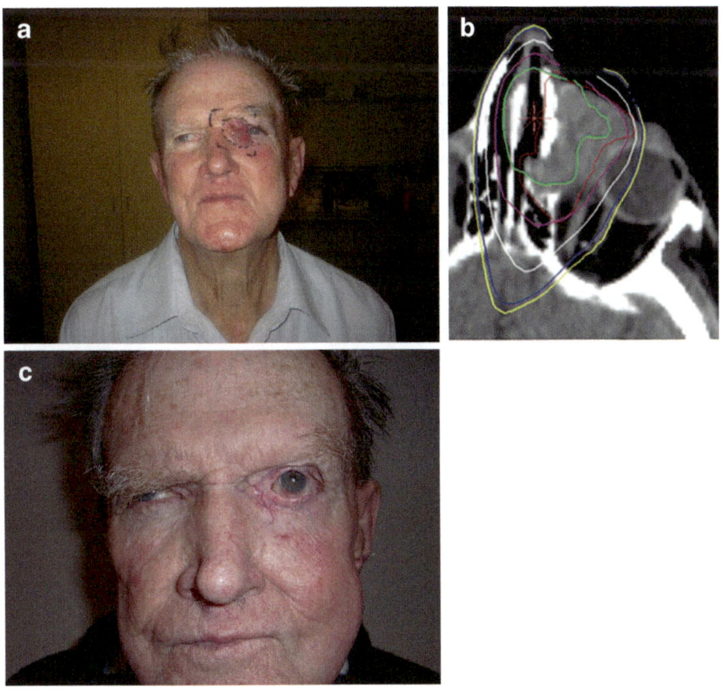

Fig. 7.3 (**a**) Cooperative 70-year-old man with only one eye with vision, with a medial canthus cSCC in that eye has recurred despite four separate operations for clearance. (**b**) Axial CT slice showing tumour invading medial wall of orbit with dosimetry. Note that the anterior chamber of the eye moved laterally to decrease dose. (**c**) Photo taken 30 months post-RT in complete remission and still able to read a newspaper

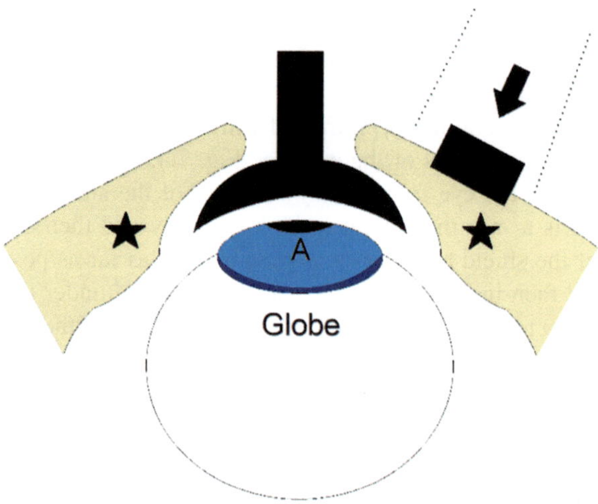

Fig. 7.4 Traditional internal eye shield (IES). "A" refers to the anterior chamber of the eye which is RT sensitive. "Globe" refers to the eye globe. The stars indicate upper and lower eyelids. On the right-sided eyelid, there is a skin lesion requiring SXRT represented as a black rectangle. This is being irradiated by the incident beam shown by the black arrow. Dotted lines show the lateral extent of the beam. The large black device above the anterior chamber is the IES. Note that the IES rests on cornea, which is the surface of the radiation-sensitive anterior chamber. The IES protects the anterior chamber when the eye is in a neutral position. Note that the IES handle parts the eyelids and protrudes above the level of the eyelids beyond the body contour, which needs to be avoided by the patient and RT staff. There is also a risk of collision with the SXRT applicator. If this occurs, there is a risk of eye trauma, and a repeat calibration of the treatment set-up may be required

The Eyelid as an RT Organ at Risk (OAR)

The eyelid is an OAR when it is inadvertently included in the radiation volume, which is centred on another nearby tissue. Examples include external beam radical PORT aimed at the maxillary sinus. In this case, the eyes are treated open in order to retract the superior eyelid away from the beam, thereby reducing the chance of epilation of the dominant superior eyelashes. Another example is palliative megavoltage photon RT to choroidal metastases with a direct anterior portal through the anterior of the globe. The eyes are treated open so that the closed eyelids do not create a bolus effect, which would increase the dose to the anterior structures. When treating pterygium with strontium-90 plaque brachytherapy, the plaque has a backing that absorbs the dose that would enter the eyelid.

Dose

The dose and treatment scheme are discussed in the general sections (Chap. 5). Fractionated treatment regimens are recommended to reduce radiation side effects and may produce better cosmetic outcomes.

Treatment-Related Side Effects

Acute Effects

These side effects are treated on a symptomatic basis. They include acute effects in skin such as skin erythema, epilation, and dry and moist desquamation and in the conjunctivae such as erythema and radiation conjunctivitis. The latter can predispose to infection, and prophylactic topical antibiotics such as chloromycetin eye drops and ointment can be administered. Acute conjunctivitis is common with doses of 30 Gy.

Blockage of the naso-lacrimal duct can occur when the medial eyelids, especially the inferior eyelid, are treated to a radical dose, and the resulting fibrosis can block the naso-lacrimal duct causing epiphora. Referral for surgical recanalization by an ophthalmologist may be necessary.

Late Effects

Xerophthalmia, the major side effect following RT to the eyelids, is irritating and may ultimately result in a non-seeing eye due to corneal opacity and a request for enucleation, and so it needs to be avoided. Xerophthalmia may occur as a result of damage to either inner eyelid surface glands, meibomian glands, or lacrimal gland acinar cells [7]. Dysfunction of the meibomian gland results in tear oil deficiency and in severe cases may lead to corneal desiccation. With conventional fractionation, the probability of xerophthalmia within 5 years of treatment is 5% (TD 5/5) and 50% (TD 50/5) [8, 9] with 35 Gy and 50 Gy, respectively, to the ocular surface [10]. The tolerance dose of TD 5/5 represents the radiation dose that would result in 5% risk of severe complications within 5 years after irradiation, and TD 50/5 represents the dose that would result in 50% probability of developing severe complications within 5 years after irradiation.

In practice, it is important to avoid irradiating all of both eyelids to prevent resting xerophthalmia. Try to keep half of each eyelid to less than these doses to preserve resting lubrication. Xerophthalmia is treated with ocular lubricants, artificial tear drops, and anti-inflammatory agents. Pre-RT ophthalmological review is recommended if post-RT effects are expected [7].

Conjunctival telangiectasia is a benign vascular change in the conjunctiva that typically occurs at doses exceeding 30 Gy. RT doses of 35 Gy have resulted in a significant incidence of late complications at the ocular surface in patients treated for orbital lymphoma [1]. Hypofractionation on the eyelids is discouraged as it leads to greater late term fibrosis.

Chronic conjunctivitis, squamous metaplasia, and conjunctival keratinization formation have been reported after doses exceeding 50 Gy [7].

Damage to the anterior structures of the eyes is avoided with appropriate shielding and planning. If they cannot be avoided, the lens is particularly prone to cataract formation with doses as low as 4 Gy. The time of onset is dose related. The threshold dose for retinal damage is usually considered to be 30–35 Gy. TD 5/5 of the retina is estimated to be 45–50 Gy, and TD 50/5 is 55 Gy [8]. The risk of radiation retinopathy is increased by coexistent diabetic retinopathy.

References

1. Wang L, Shan Y, Dai X, You N, Shao J, Pan X, Gao T, Ye J. Clinicopathological analysis of 5146 eyelid tumours and tumour-like lesions in an eye centre in South China, 2000–2018: a retrospective cohort study. BMJ Open. 2021;11(1):e041854.
2. Petsuksiri J, Frank SJ, Garden AS, Ang KK, Morrison WH, Chao KS, Rosenthal DI, Schwartz DL, Ahamad A, Esmaeli B. Outcomes after radiotherapy for squamous cell carcinoma of the eyelid. Cancer. 2008;112(1):111–8.
3. Fogarty LM, Fogarty GB, Hong A, Scolyer RA, Lin E, Haydu L, Guitera P, Thompson J. Radiotherapy for lentigo maligna: a literature review and recommendations for treatment. Br J Dermatol. 2014;170(1):52–8.
4. Takagawa Y, Tamaki W, Suzuki S, Inaba K, Murakami N, Takahashi K, Igaki H, Nakayama Y, Shigematsu N, Itami J. Radiotherapy for localized sebaceous carcinoma of the eyelid: a retrospective analysis of 83 patients. J Radiat Res. 2019;60(5):622–9.
5. Hata M, Koike I, Omura M, Maegawa J, Ogino I, Inoue T. Noninvasive and curative radiation therapy for sebaceous carcinoma of the eyelid. Int J Radiat Oncol Biol Phys. 2012;82(2):605–11.
6. Gorjiara T, Conway A, Sullivan J, et al. A technique for external beam radiotherapy to the eyelid without the need for an internal eye shield. Int J Radiol Radiat Ther. 2021;8(3):92–8.
7. Akagunduz OO, Yilmaz SG, Tavlayan E, Baris ME, Afrashi F, Esassolak M. Radiation-induced ocular surface disorders and retinopathy: ocular structures and radiation dose-volume effect. Cancer Res Treat. 2022;54(2):417–23.
8. Emami B, Lyman J, Brown A, Coia L, Goiten M, Munzenride JE, et al. Tolerance of normal tissue to therapeutic radiation. Int J Radiat Oncol Biol Phys. 1991;21:109–22.
9. Rubin P, Cassarett G. A direction for clinical radiation pathology. In: Vaeth JM, et al., editors. Frontiers of radiation therapy and oncology VI. Baltimore: University Park Press; 1972. p. 1–16.
10. Durkin SR, Roos D, Higgs B, Casson RJ, Selva D. Ophthalmic and adnexal complications of radiotherapy. Acta Ophthalmol Scand. 2007;85(3):240–50.

Chapter 8
Lip

Romaana Mir and Agata Rembielak

The lips surround the oral aperture (Fig. 8.1). In the central region, the superior border corresponds to the inferior margin of the base of the nose. The lateral limit of the lip follows the alar sulci; the upper and lower lips join at the lateral commissure. The inferior limit of the lips in the central region is the mentolabial sulcus. The philtrum and pillars are part of the upper lip.

The surface of the lip is comprised of four zones: hairy skin, vermilion border, vermilion, and oral mucosa.

The Union for International Cancer Control (UICC) and the American Joint Committee on Cancer (AJCC) TNM Eighth Edition Head and Neck and Skin classification categorise the lip into anatomical subsites:

Lip	External upper lip (vermilion border) (C00.00)
	External lower lip (vermilion border) (C00.1)
	Commissures (C00.6)
	Lip (excluding vermilion surface) (C44.0)
Buccal mucosa	Mucosa of upper lip (C00.3)
	Mucosa of lower lip (C00.4)
	Cheek mucosa (C06.0)

R. Mir
Mount Vernon Cancer Centre, Northwood, UK

The Univeristy of Manchester, Manchester, UK
e-mail: romaana.mir@nhs.net

A. Rembielak (✉)
Department of Clinical Oncology, The Christie NHS Foundation Trust, Manchester, UK

Division of Cancer Sciences, School of Medical Sciences, Faculty of Biology, Medicine and Health, The University of Manchester, Manchester, UK
e-mail: agata.rembielak@nhs.net

K. J. Joseph et al. (eds.), *Radiotherapy in Skin Cancer*,
https://doi.org/10.1007/978-3-031-44316-9_8

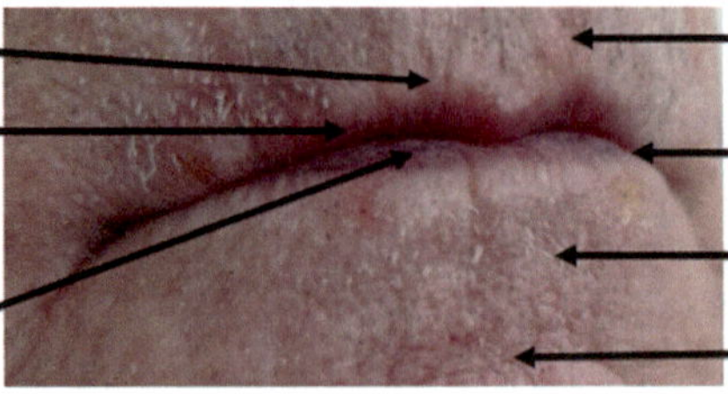

Fig. 8.1 Anatomy and landmarks of the lip

Carcinoma of the lip accounts for 25% of oral carcinomas. 82% of lip carcinomas develop on the lower lip, 10% at the upper lip, and 8% at the lateral commissure [1].

The incidence of lip carcinoma is 3–12/100,000 with predominance in geographical regions with high ultraviolet exposure, in those who are smokers, and in males over 50 years of age [2, 3]. Smoking along with immunosuppression is a prognostic risk factor; case series identifies advancing age as a factor associated with poorer outcomes and more aggressive disease.

Given the high visibility of the lip, most lip carcinomas are detected early. Recurrence rates range from 5–35% and are dependent on tumour size, location, previous treatment, and primary pathology [4]. The mortality associated with large or recurrent lip carcinoma is reported in up to 15% [5]; in cases of local lymph node involvement, the 5-year mortality is up to 50% [6].

The behaviour of lip carcinomas is distinct from carcinomas of the oral cavity and are primarily managed as a cutaneous carcinoma; tumour board discussion with surgeons and radiation oncology colleagues who manage primary head and neck carcinomas is advised for complex cases.

Cutaneous squamous cell carcinoma (cSCC) predominates at the lower lip (67%), whereas basal cell carcinoma (BCC) is more frequent at the upper lip (56%) and philtrum (67%). Synchronous dysplasia is evident in half of the lip cSCC with synchronous cSCC seen in 5%.

The incidence of lip carcinoma metastasis to cervical lymph nodes is 5–20%, with cervical level Ia/b involvement most common [7]. Prophylactic neck dissection is not recommended for early-stage disease; ultrasound of the draining lymph nodes is appropriate for surveillance of the clinically negative neck. Lymph node metastases are rarely seen in BCC.

Surgery is regarded as the main treatment modality; radiotherapy (RT) should be considered to preserve function and cosmesis, for inoperable tumours, in instances with multiple lesions, and in the post-operative setting for adjuvant management of high-risk features and lymph node involvement. Primary radical RT and surgery are equal treatment options for early-stage T1–T2 carcinoma, where both achieve excellent local control [3]. Like carcinomas of the nose, cure with preservation of function and cosmesis is the fundamental consideration in the treatment recommendation.

Australian case series describe improved outcomes with primary surgery followed by adjuvant RT in instances of positive or close excision margins (≤2 mm); recurrence-free survival is 51% with surgery alone and 92% with surgery followed by adjuvant RT ($p = 0.008$) [8].

This chapter discusses external beam RT for lip carcinoma.

Indications for Radiotherapy

Primary RT is offered to patients with all stages of carcinoma of lip, particularly for elderly patients who may not be suitable for radical surgery due to medical comorbidities.

Adjuvant RT is considered post-operatively for [6, 9–12]
- T3–T4 disease
- Residual disease after surgery
- Close* or positive pathological margin
- Perineural and/or lymphovascular space invasion
- Presence of two or more risk factors including tumour diameter >2 cm, poor differentiation, and tumour thickness ≥4 mm

*The definition of close pathological margin differs among recommendations and is referred to as <2 mm or <1 mm.

Treatment Approach

The lip is a flat surface with minimal tissue inhomogeneities and can be treated with either orthovoltage photons or electrons. Volumetric modulated arc therapy (VMAT) delivery is an option for larger treatment volumes but may result in low-dose bath to the alveolar ridge, mandible, and oral cavity; dose and ensuant toxicity to these structures can be avoided with RT delivery via a direct field.

Treatment Planning

Radiotherapy treatment techniques for lip carcinoma
- Orthovoltage (Fig. 8.2)
- Electrons (Fig. 8.3)
- Intensity-modulated radiation therapy (IMRT)/VMAT (Fig. 8.4)

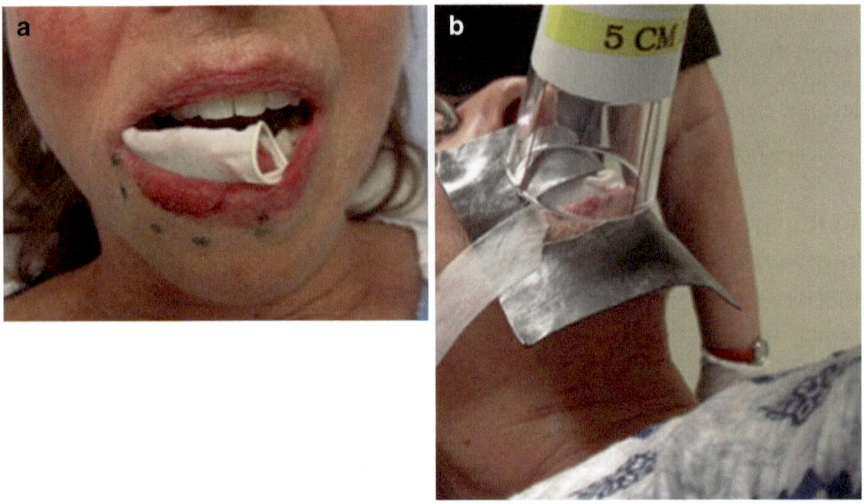

Fig. 8.2 Cutaneous SCC of the lower lip treated with primary radical orthovoltage 200 kVp 50 Gy in 20 daily fractions. (**a**) Radiotherapy planning with delineated treatment volume and intraoral shield. (**b**) Custom-made lead cut-out with 5 cm cone. Images courtesy of Dr. Toni Barnes

Target Volume

In the radical setting, the target volume encompasses the primary tumour with additional margins for clinical target volume (CTV), planning target volume (PTV), and departmental electron field penumbra when RT is delivered with electrons. The peripheral margin from tumour edge to field edge is commonly 10 mm for orthovoltage and larger at 15–20 mm with electrons to allow for the field penumbra at depth.

In the adjuvant setting, the target volume is considered in view of the preoperative extent of carcinoma, operative approach and reconstruction, and surgical scar. The PTV and, where applicable, the departmental electron field penumbra margins apply; the CTV margin may be omitted in view of the adequacy of the peripheral surgical margin.

In both the radical and adjuvant settings, the target volume is delineated clinically. If it is not possible to confidently measure the thickness of the tumour or the lip, a CT slice can be taken for depth measurement.

Treatment Set-Up and Field Arrangement

The patient is positioned supine in a comfortable, reproducible position. The lip is examined under a bright light and the treatment field from tumour edge or scar to radiotherapy field edge is delineated by a certified radiation oncologist.

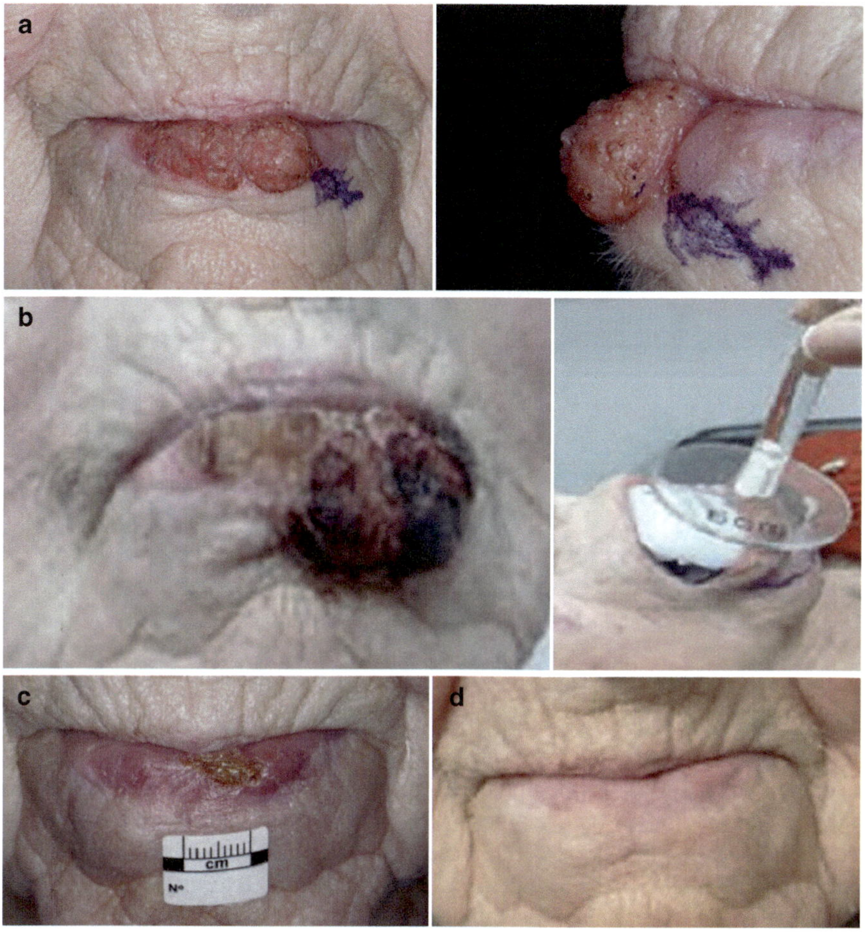

Fig. 8.3 Cutaneous SCC of the lower lip treated with primary radical radiotherapy 12 MeV electrons 40 Gy in 8 daily fractions. (**a**) First presentation. (**b**) Radiotherapy planning with intraoral shield. (**c**) 2-Month follow-up. (**d**) 6-Month follow-up

The thickness of the lip at the central axis defines the orthovoltage or electron beam energy, which is commonly 200 kVp or 6–9 MeV. The electron beam incident isodose and exit dose at the inner surface of the lip should be greater than or equal to 90%; to achieve 90% incident isodose, tissue equivalent bolus is applied to the skin surface to manipulate the electron beam to enable delivery of therapeutic RT dose to the target volume. The orthovoltage incident dose is 100%, negating the requirement for tissue equivalent bolus.

In both the radical and adjuvant settings, a wax-covered intraoral lead shield is placed in the space behind the mucosal surface of the lip and in front of the teeth to stop the RT beam and subsequent dose delivery to the alveolar ridge, mandible, and oral cavity. The thickness of the lead is proportional to the beam energy and much

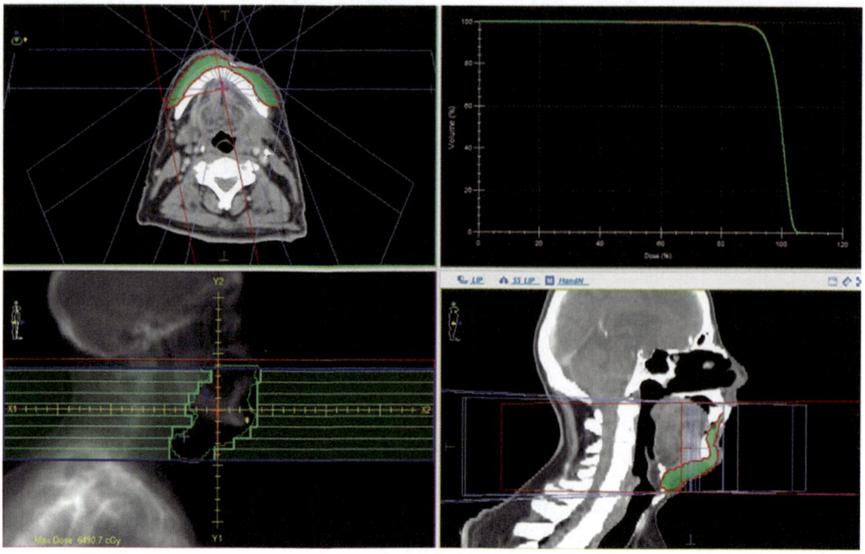

Fig. 8.4 pT3N0M0 cSCC of the lower lip treated with IMRT 6MV 60 Gy in 30 daily fractions over 6 weeks. Green contour PTV60. Images courtesy of Mrs. Anysja Zuchora

thinner for orthovoltage treatment, which is typically 3–4 mm thick. The wax covering limits backscatter to the inner surface of the lip; without the wax, the dose delivery to the inner surface of the lip is 30–50% over the expected prescribed dose. In the adjuvant setting, post-surgical loss of tissue and fibrosis may limit the available space between the lip and teeth; in these instances placement of the wax-covered intraoral lead shield can be a challenge.

The alveolar ridge, mandible, and nasal septum are organs at risk. The alveolar ridge and mandible are shielded by the intraoral shield. The position of the lip carcinoma or surgical scar may occasionally result in the base of the nasal septum being encompassed within the treatment field; the radiation oncologist will discuss the risks and benefits of unintended nasal septum irradiation with the patient in advance of treatment delivery.

Elective Nodal Irradiation

For high-risk lip carcinomas, selected institutions deliver 50 Gy elective nodal irradiation to the first echelon lymph nodes as an alternative to prophylactic neck dissection; with this approach, the rate of isolated recurrence within electively irradiated lymph nodes is 2.8% [13]. Randomised data are not available, therefore elective lymph node irradiation is not currently considered as standard of care but may be considered on a case-by-case basis for high-risk primary lip carcinomas.

Dose

The principles and overview of dose and treatment schedules for skin carcinoma are discussed in earlier chapters.

Hypofractionated schedules have an application in older patients where prompt gain of tumour control is balanced against the frequency of hospital visits and the incidence of late effects. There is no specific dose fractionation recommended for the lip; the schedules most used in the radical or adjuvant setting are [14]:

- 40–45 Gy in 8–10 fractions over 2 weeks
- 50–55 Gy 15–20 fractions over 3–4 weeks
- 60 Gy in 30 fractions over 6 weeks

Treatment-Related Side Effects

The common acute side effects are
- Tiredness
- Skin redness, soreness, swelling, bleeding
- Ulceration of the lip and lip/oral mucosa
- Reduced oral intake
- Requirement for analgesia

The late side effects following lip RT are
- Thicker or thinner skin
- Hypo-or hyperpigmentation of the skin
- Permanent hair loss
- Telangiectasia
- Fibrosis

Palliative Radiotherapy

Palliative RT is recommended when there are no viable curative options. The hypofractionated regimes used in palliative RT for lip carcinoma are the same as in other skin carcinoma sites:

- 12–20 Gy in 1 fraction
- 14.8 Gy in 4 fractions twice daily over 2 consecutive days (QUAD shot, also used in re-irradiation) [15]
- 20 Gy in 2 fractions 1 week apart
- 30 Gy in 10 fractions over 2 weeks
- 35 Gy in 5 fractions 3 times per week
- 8 Gy per fraction delivered on days 0, 7, and 21

Outcomes

Primary radical RT achieves greater than 80% local control and cure in early-stage lip carcinoma [2, 3, 8, 16–19]. The local in-field failure rate is 4.6–5%; isolated in-field failure is best managed with salvage surgery [16, 17].

Tumour thickness greater than 4 mm, perineural invasion, or close or positive margins are high-risk features; in these circumstances, the best outcomes are achieved with surgery followed by post-operative RT.

As local control outcomes with primary surgery or primary radical RT in early-stage lip carcinoma are equivocal, prospective measurement of patient-reported outcome measures and quality-of-life metrics are required. The long-term outcome measures quantifying cosmesis, function, and morbidity will help guide patients to make an informed decision regarding their lip carcinoma treatment.

References

1. Hu C-Y, Pan Z-Y, Yang J, Chu X-H, Zhang J, Tao X-J, Chen W-M, Li Y-J, Lyu J. Nomograms for predicting long-term overall survival and cancer-specific survival in lip squamous cell carcinoma: a population-based study. Cancer Med. 2019;8:4032–42.
2. Gooris PFF, Maat B, Vermey A, Roukema JA, Roodenburg JLN. Radiotherapy for cancer of the lip: a long-term evaluation of 85 treated cases. Oral Surg Oral Med Oral Pathol Radiol Endod. 1998;86:325–30.
3. McCombe D, MacGill K, Ainslie J, Beresford J, Matthew J. Squamous cell carcinoma of the lip: a retrospective review of the Peter MacCallum Cancer Institute experience 1979–1988. Aust NZJ Surg. 2000;70:358–61.
4. Agostini T, Spinelli G, Arcuri F, Perello R. Metastatic squamous cell carcinoma of the lower lip: analysis of the 5-year survival rate. Arch Craniofac Surg. 2017;18:105–11.
5. Veness MJ, Ong C, Cakir B, Morgan G. Squamous cell carcinoma of the lip. Patterns of relapse and outcome: reporting the Westmead Hospital experience 1980–1997. Australas Radiol. 2001;45:195–9.
6. Likhacheva A, Awan M, Barker CA, Bhatnagar A, Bradfield L, Brady MS, Buzurovic I, Geiger JL, Parvathaneni U, Zaky S, Devlin PM. Definitive and postoperative radiation therapy for basal and squamous cell cancers of the skin: executive summary of an American Society for Radiation Oncology clinical practice guideline. Pract Radiat Oncol. 2020;10:8–20.
7. Gooris PJJ, Vermey A, de Visscher JGAM, Burlage FR, Roodenburg JLN. Supraomohyoid neck dissection in the management of cervical lymph node metastases of squamous cell carcinoma of the lower lip. Head Neck. 2002;24:678–83.
8. Najim M, Cross S, Gebski V, Palme CE, Morgan GJ, Veness MJ. Early-stage squamous cell carcinoma of the lip: the Australian experience and the benefits of radiotherapy in improving outcome in high-risk patients after resection. Head Neck. 2013;35:1426–30.
9. Keohane SG, Botting J, Budny PG, Dolan OM, Fife K, Harwood CA, Mallipeddi R, Marsden JR, Motley RJ, Newlands C, Proby C, Rembielak A, Slater DN, Smithson JA, Buckley P, Fairbrother P, Hashme M, Mustapa MFM, Exton LS, on behalf of the British Association of Dermatologists' Clinical Standards Unit. British Association of Dermatologists guidelines for the management of people with cutaneous squamous cell carcinoma 2020. Br J Dermatol. 2021;184:401–14.

10. Nasr I, McGrath EJ, Harwood CA, Botting J, Buckley P, Budny PG, Fairbrother P, Fife K, Gupta G, Hashme M, Hoey S, Lear JT, Mallipeddi R, Mallon E, Motley RJ, Newlands C, Newman J, Pynn EV, Shroff N, Slater DN, Exton LS, Mustapa MFM, Ezejimofor MC, On behalf of the British Association of Dermatologists' Clinical Standards Unit. British Association of Dermatologists guidelines for the management of adults with basal cell carcinoma 2021. Br J Dermatol. 2021;185:899–920.
11. Peris K, Fargnoli MC, Garbe C, Kaufmann R, Bastholt L, Seguin NB, Bataille V, Del Marmol V, Dummer R, Harwood CA, Hauschild A, Holler C, Haedersdal M, Malvehy J, Middleton MR, Morton CA, Nagore E, Stratigos AJ, Szeimies R-M, Tagliaferri L, Trakatelli M, Zalaudek I, Eggermont A, Grob JJ, On Behalf of European Dermatology Forum (EDF), the European Association of Dermato-Oncology (EADO) and the European Organization for Research and Treatment of Cancer (EORTC). Diagnosis and treatment of basal cell carcinoma: European consensus-based interdisciplinary guidelines. Eur J Cancer. 2019;118:10–34.
12. Stratigos AJ, Garbe C, Dessinioti C, Lebbe C, Bataille V, Bastholt L, Dreno B, Fargnoli MC, Forsea AM, Frenard C, Harwood CA, Hauschild A, Hoeller C, Kandolf-Sekulovic L, Kaufmann R, Kelleners-Smeets NMJ, Malvehy J, del Marmol V, Middleton MR, Moreno-Ramirez D, Pellecani G, Peris K, Saiag P, van den Beuken-van Everdingen MHJ, Vieira R, Zalaudek I, Eggermont AMM, Grob JJ, On Behalf of the European Dermatology Forum (EDF), the European Association of Dermato-Oncology (EADO) and the European Organization for Research and Treatment of Cancer (EORTC). European interdisciplinary guideline on invasive squamous cell carcinoma of the skin: part 2. Treatment. Eur J Cancer. 2020;128:83–102.
13. Wray J, Amdur RJ, Morris CG, Werning J, Mendenhall WM. Efficacy of elective nodal irradiation in skin squamous cell carcinoma of the face, ears, and scalp. Radiat Oncol. 2015;10:199.
14. McPartlin AJ, Slevin NJ, Sykes AJ, Rembielak A. Radiotherapy treatment of non-melanoma skin cancer: a survey of current UK practice and commentary. Br J Radiol. 2014;87:20140501.
15. Vuong W, Lin J, Wei RL. Palliative radiotherapy for skin malignancies. Ann Palliat Med. 2017;6:165–72.
16. Corry J, Peters LJ, Costa ID, Milner AD, Fawns H, Rischin D, Porceddu S. The 'QUAD SHOT'—a phase II study of palliative radiotherapy for incurable head and neck cancer. Radiother Oncol. 2005;77(2):137–42.
17. de Visscher JGAM, Grond AJK, Botke G, van der Waal I. Results of radiotherapy in squamous cell carcinoma of the vermilion border of the lower lip. A retrospective analysis of 108 patients. Radiother Oncol. 1996;39:9–14.
18. Pham TT, Cross S, Gebski V, Veness MJ. Squamous cell carcinoma of the lip in Australian patients: definitive radiotherapy is an efficacious option to surgery in select patients. Dermatol Surg. 2015;41:219–25.
19. Piccinno R, Tavecchio S, Benzecry V. Superficial radiotherapy for non-melanoma skin cancer of the lip: a 44-year Italian experience. J Dermatol Treat. 2020;31:382–6.

Chapter 9
Ear

Elizabeth A. Barnes and May N. Tsao

Introduction

Basal cell carcinoma (BCC) and cutaneous squamous cell carcinoma (cSCC) are collectively referred to as keratinocyte carcinomas (KCs) and are the most common cancers diagnosed worldwide. They are found predominantly in the sun-exposed regions such as the head and neck, with 6–10% of KC located on the ear [1]. The ear is a high-risk anatomical location for locoregional recurrence. Lesions in the crevices and posterior pinna may have delayed diagnosis as these locations are not readily visible. The external ear consists of the pinna (auricle) and external auditory canal which terminates at the tympanic membrane. When the tumor extends into the external auditory canal, assessment by a head and neck surgeon and radiation oncologist is warranted due to the risk of subclinical extension into the canal. This chapter is limited to discussion of KC involving the pinna. The anatomy of the pinna is complex. There is a lack of subcutaneous adipose tissue, and skin often directly overlies cartilage. Depending on the location and size of the tumor, surgery for the primary lesion may involve wedge resection or excision with skin graft. The risk of nodal metastases is >10% for high-risk cSCC; therefore, CT imaging, with consideration for sentinel lymph nodal assessment, may be warranted in select cases [2].

E. A. Barnes (✉) · M. N. Tsao
Odette Cancer Centre, University of Toronto, Toronto, ON, Canada
e-mail: toni.barnes@sunnybrook.ca

K. J. Joseph et al. (eds.), *Radiotherapy in Skin Cancer*,
https://doi.org/10.1007/978-3-031-44316-9_9

Indications for Radiotherapy

RT can be used in the definitive, adjuvant, and palliative setting. For definitive management of KC, the major advantage of RT over surgery is the ability to preserve function and cosmesis. Regarding function, wedge resection may remove a large portion of the helix, resulting in difficulty wearing glasses. Distortion of the conchal bowel can cause issues with placement of hearing aids. Cosmesis may be impaired when surgery removes a portion of the helix, resulting in facial asymmetry.

In the adjuvant setting, RT may be utilized when risk factors for local recurrence are present. cSCC tends to be more aggressive than BCC. Risk factors for considering postoperative RT (PORT) for cSCC include close or positive margins when further surgery is not possible, a T3 or 4 lesion, and the setting of recurrence. Adjuvant RT of the nodal bed is recommended in the postoperative setting for positive node(s), except for a solitary <3 cm node with no extracapsular invasion. Including the undissected regional nodal bed for high-risk cSCC tumors (i.e., thickness >6 mm) may be considered when treatment of the primary site overlaps, such as the parotid or upper cervical region [3]. For BCC, PORT may be considered in similar clinical scenarios; however, the strength of recommendation is lower, and given the very low risk of nodal metastases with BCC, elective nodal RT is not recommended [3].

Palliative RT can offer symptom palliation for bleeding, discharge, pain, and odor for KC on the pinna.

Treatment Approach

The irregular surface contour of the pinna makes treatment planning challenging. External beam treatment modalities include kilovoltage, electrons, and photons [either with parallel opposed or wedge pair technique, and intensity-modulated radiation therapy (IMRT) or volumetric modulated arc therapy (VMAT)]. Brachytherapy with a custom surface applicator for superficial tumors (<5 mm deep) or interstitial technique for deeper tumors (>5 mm) is an option for delivering conformal treatment and is beyond the scope of this chapter. Considerations for choosing the optimal treatment modality include tumor factors such as location, size, depth, and nearby organs at risk (OAR); patient factors including tolerance for radiation setup; and availability of modality at the treating center.

The advantages and disadvantage of these external beam modalities are summarized in Table 9.1.

Table 9.1 Common advantages and disadvantages of external beam treatment modalities for the pinna

	Advantages	Disadvantages
Kilovoltage	Ease of planning (clinical markup with pen)	Target needs to be flat
	Ease of setup (clinical)	High f-factor (cartilage and bone) with low energies
	Ease of treatment (no need for image verification or custom immobilization, patient can be treated sitting in chair)	May require shielding
	No need for bolus as the surface dose is 100%	Kilovoltage machines not available in all centers
	Narrow penumbra leading to smaller field sizes (compared to electrons and photons) resulting in sparing of organs and risk and ability to hypofractionate	
Electrons	Rapid dose falloff with depth	Minimum field size (4–5 cm^2) required
	Clinical markup possible for well-defined lesions	Bolus required to achieve full skin dose
		Tissue equivalent material required to fill conchal bowel and ensure flat target surface
		Larger penumbra (up to 1 cm) compared to kilovoltage
		Lower relative biological effectiveness (RBE) than kilovoltage and photons
Photons	Useful for larger, deep-seated tumors, and covering elective nodal bed	Bolus required to achieve full skin dose
	CT planning allows for target and organ-at-risk delineation	Custom immobilization required
		CT simulation and planning required
		Daily imaging verification required for IMRT/VMAT
		Increased-volume low-dose radiation delivered outside of target volume with IMRT/VMAT, i.e., larger area hair loss

Treatment Planning

To help decide the optimal treatment modality, it is often helpful to clinically delineate on the pinna the gross tumor volume (GTV), with the appropriate clinical target volume (CTV) (5–10 mm depending on histology and tumor size). The PTV margin depends on patient immobilization.

If the resultant target volume is <10 mm thick, and on a flat surface where the applicator cone can approximate the skin so "standoff" is not an issue, kilovoltage may be considered. The penumbra for orthovoltage is narrow (2 mm), which results in a comparatively smaller field size. The ease of planning and simple setup (the cone applicator is pressed against the patient's skin and helps immobilize the patient) and treatment (no need for bolus) make this an ideal modality to treat frail, elderly patients. Also, patients can be treated sitting or on a stretcher and do not have to be transferred to a treatment couch.

For larger (>4–5 cm) and thicker targets, electrons with the appropriate use of tissue equivalent material (bolus) may be preferred. Wax is used to fill the conchal bowl "earplug" to create a flat surface and can be placed posterior to the pinna to fill any air gaps. Tissue equivalent bolus (0.5–1 cm) such as superflab is often required overtop to ensure full skin dose. A wire mesh bolus of high-atomic-number material can also be used to achieve full skin dose. At the time of treatment planning, target volumes are drawn clinically on the patient, electron field size is chosen, template is made, and photographs are taken as a reference of the target volume and bolus placements. Lead shielding behind the pinna can be used to reduce exit dose. The choice of electron energy can be made by measuring tumor thickness clinically, and the dose is calculated manually. CT planning to model electron distribution can also be done. However, lead shielding cannot be used during CT simulation.

When delivering a uniform dose to the target volume while respecting dose to OAR (i.e., cochlea) with electrons is not feasible, and for larger more deeply seated tumors or when nodal coverage is required, CT planning usually with photons is used. Superficial tumors are difficult to visualize on CT images, and the target volume (GTV and/or CTV) should be wired at the time of simulation to aid visualization. MRI simulation may be considered for deeper tumors to aid in target delineation. A thermoplastic mask is made for immobilization and to facilitate reproducible bolus placement. Stereotactic body radiotherapy (SBRT) with dose escalation over standard palliative dosing can be considered for medically unfit patients with the goal of improving local control [4].

Examples to illustrate these three external beam modalities are shown below. Of note, for the electron distribution shown in Fig. 9.3b, our planning system does not use Monte Carlo and as such the electron distribution shown is not accurate especially for isodoses less than 80%. The distribution shown also does not account for tissue inhomogeneity.

Case 1 1.5 cm BCC on the left posterior pinna extending to helical rim, 1 cm margin from GTV to field edge given. Treated with 180 kV orthovoltage, 3.5 cm circle, and lead shielding anterior to pinna to block exit dose (Fig. 9.1a, b).

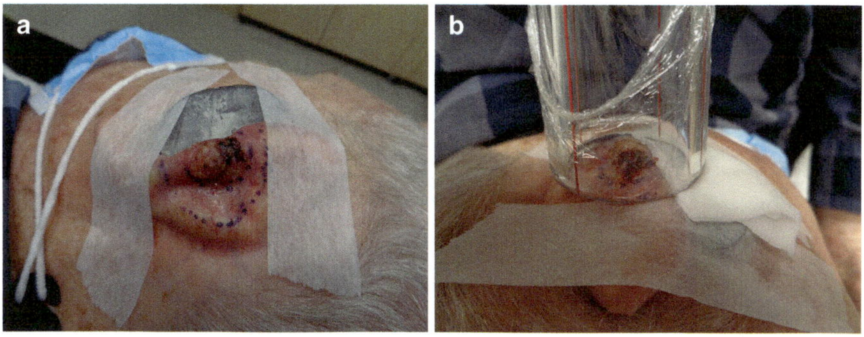

Fig. 9.1 (**a**, **b**) BCC treated with orthovoltage. (**a**) Treatment setup showing GTV, field edge, and lead shielding anterior to pinna. (**b**) Conical applicator covering target

Case 2 2 cm cSCC on right posterior pinna extending to scalp, regional lymph nodes uninvolved. Treated with VMAT technique, 50 Gy in 20 fractions (Fig. 9.2a–c).

Case 3 2.5 cm BCC right superior pinna (Fig. 9.3a, b).

Dose

The dose fractionation regimens for KC of the pinna are similar for KC in other sites. Conventionally fractionated regimens are delivered in 2 Gy per fraction for a total dose of 60–66 Gy. RT for KC is often hypofractionated due to the smaller field size, lack of critical structures, and goal of facilitating treatment delivery for the often frail and elderly patient population. Hypofractionated treatment can be delivered in 1–4 fractions per week. A 2017 meta-analysis suggested using regimens with a $BED_3 = 100$ Gy such as 50 Gy/15 fr, 36.75 Gy/7 fr, or 35 Gy/5 fr as they resulted in "good" cosmesis in 80% of patients [5].

Hypofractionated regimens for KC on the pinna, especially using kilovoltage with the high f-factor, may be of concern to practitioners due to the risk of cartilage and bone necrosis. Rates of necrosis are reported as 0–13% [6–9], with most healing with conservative management. Associated risk factors for necrosis were found to include dose per fraction [6, 7] suggested to be kept <4 Gy particularly for field sizes >5 cm^2 in one series where orthovoltage was used in 83% of patients [6], and >6 Gy per fraction and treatment time <5 days where both electrons (43%) and orthovoltage (57%) were used [7].

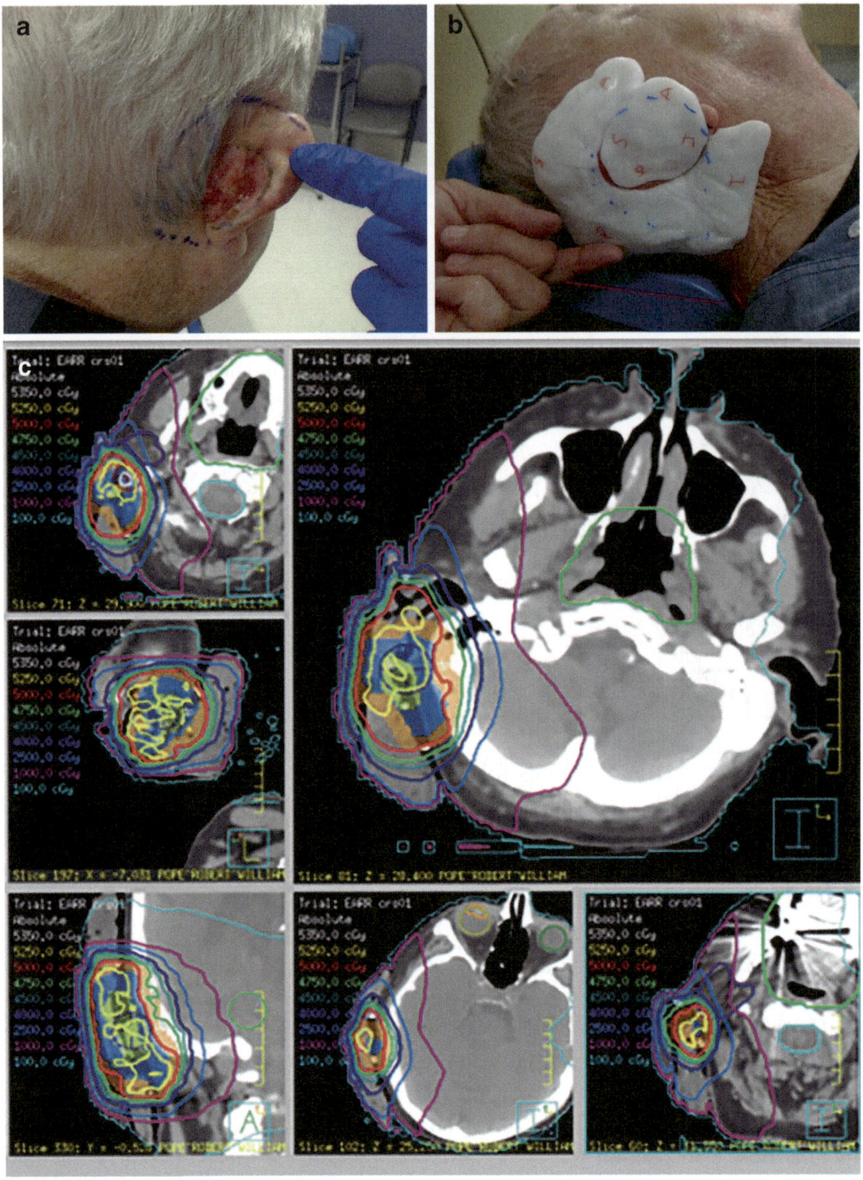

Fig. 9.2 (**a**–**c**) cSCC on posterior pinna treated with VMAT. (**a**) GTV and CTV marked. (**b**) Tissue equivalent bolus filling conchal bowel and surrounding pinna. (**c**) VMAT distribution, green isodose line showing 95% CTV (orange) coverage

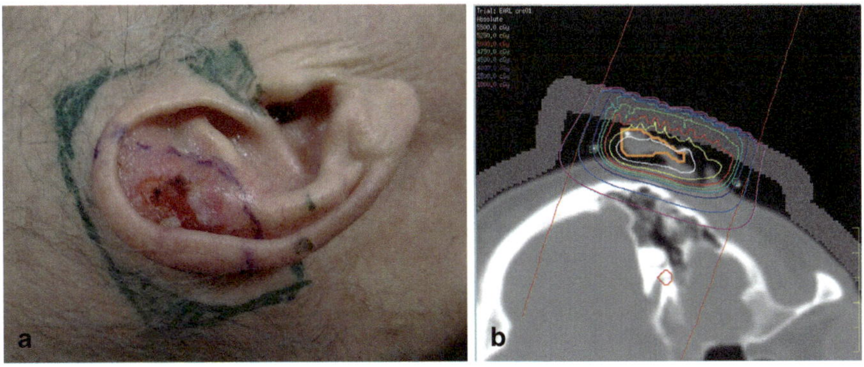

Fig. 9.3 (**a**) CTV and electron field edge marked. (**b**) 9 MeV electrons, tissue equivalent bolus (orange, yellow, white) surrounding target (bright orange), 1 cm bolus covering field, 100% red isodose line covering target volume (orange)

Treatment-Related Side Effects and Management

Acute side effects of treatment include fatigue, skin dryness, pruritus, and erythema with progression from dry to moist desquamation. Edema of the pinna with resulting discomfort can also be seen. Acute skin reactions are managed with saline soaks, topical corticosteroids, and silver sulfadiazine [10]. Late skin side effects (>3 months from treatment) can include atrophy, hypo- or hyperpigmentation, and telangiectasia. Delayed wound healing and cartilage necrosis are also risks.

Outcomes

Four series were found reporting outcomes exclusively for KC of the pinna. Five-year rates of local control are 78–93%, utilizing both kilovoltage and electron modalities [6–9]. Large tumor size and low BED were associated with local failure in one series [6].

References

1. Leiter U, Eigentler T, Garbe C. Epidemiology of skin cancer. Adv Exp Med Biol. 2014;810:120–40.
2. Wermker K, Kluwig J, Schipmann S, Klein M, Schulze HJ, Hallermann C. Prediction score for lymph node metastasis from cutaneous squamous cell carcinoma of the external ear. Eur J Surg Oncol. 2015;41(1):128–35.
3. Likhacheva A, Awan M, Barker CA, Bhatnagar A, Brady MS, Buzurovic I, et al. Definitive and postoperative radiation therapy for basal and squamous cell cancers of the skin: executive

summary of an American Society for Radiation Oncology clinical practice guideline. Pract Radiat Oncol. 2020;10(1):8–20.
4. Voruganti IS, Poon I, Husain ZA, Bayley A, Barnes EA, Zhang L, Chin L, Erler D, Higgins K, Enepekides D, Eskander A, Karam I. Stereotactic body radiotherapy for head and neck skin cancer. Radiother Oncol. 2021;165:1–7.
5. Zaorsky NG, Lee CT, Zhang E, Keith SW, Galloway TJ. Hypofractionated radiation therapy for basal and squamous cell skin cancer: a meta-analysis. Radiother Oncol. 2017;125(1):13–20. https://doi.org/10.1016/j.radonc.2017.08.011.
6. Silva JJ, Tsang RW, Panzarella T, Levin W, Wells W. Results of radiotherapy for epithelial skin cancer of the pinna: the Princess Margaret Hospital experience, 1982–1993. Int J Radiat Oncol Biol Phys. 2000;47(2):451–9.
7. Hayter CR, Lee KH, Groome PA, Brundage M. Necrosis following radiotherapy for carcinoma of the pinna. Int J Radiat Oncol Biol Phys. 1996;36(5):1033–7.
8. Spigariolo CB, Berti E, Brambilla R, Piccinno R. Radiation therapy of non-melanoma skin cancer of the pinna: an Italian 35-year experience. Ital J Dermatol Venerol. 2022;157(1):92–100.
9. Caccialanza M, Piccinno R, Kolesnikova L, Gnecchi L. Radiotherapy of skin carcinomas of the pinna: a study of 115 lesions in 108 patients. Int J Dermatol. 2005;44(6):513–7.
10. Finkelstein S, Kanee L, Behroozian T, Wolf JR, van den Hurk C, Chow E, Bonomo P. Comparison of clinical practice guidelines on radiation dermatitis: a narrative review. Support Care Cancer. 2022;30(6):4663–74.

Chapter 10
Extremities

May N. Tsao and Elizabeth A. Barnes

Basal cell cancer (BCC) and cutaneous squamous cell cancer (cSCC), also categorized as keratinocyte carcinomas (KCs), are more common than all other cancers combined [1]. The major risk factor for KC is chronic sun exposure. These skin cancers typically occur on sun-exposed areas such as the face and extremities [2, 3].

A population-based study in Queensland, Australia, included 5150 participants, of whom 74.7% ($n = 3846$) had BCCs and 25.3% ($n = 1304$) had cSCCs. Body sites were classified as head and/or neck, trunk, upper limbs and lower limbs. The authors calculated the relative tumour density (RTD) as the ratio of the proportion of tumours at the anatomical site to the proportion of skin surface area at that site. These data reveal that most KCs occur in the head and neck region [4].

For the subsite of the extremity, namely the hand site, the authors reported that the RTD was 14 times higher for cSCC than for BCC, 2.70 (95% CI, 2.33–3.07) compared to 0.19 (95% CI, 0.84–0.96), respectively. The RTD for cSCC on the upper or lower extremities was almost twice that of BCC. For BCC, there was a higher RTD on less sun-exposed sites (namely trunk) compared to cSCC. These data suggest that unclear etiological factors, other than sun exposure, are important, particularly with BCC.

For patients who present with localized extremity KC, the options of management are surgery or RT, or both. Topical therapies for superficial BCC or Bowen's disease (cutaneous squamous cell carcinoma in situ) include cryotherapy, electrodessication and curettage, topical imiquimod (for superficial BCC), and photodynamic therapy.

Targeted therapy such as vismodegib (Hedgehog signalling pathway targeting agent) is a treatment option for rare metastatic basal cell skin cancers or for locally advanced basal cell skin cancer not amenable to RT or surgery.

Cemiplimab is an immunotherapy drug which has been used to treat metastatic or locally advanced cSCC.

M. N. Tsao (✉) · E. A. Barnes
Odette Cancer Centre, University of Toronto, Toronto, ON, Canada
e-mail: may.tsao@sunnybrook.ca

K. J. Joseph et al. (eds.), *Radiotherapy in Skin Cancer*,
https://doi.org/10.1007/978-3-031-44316-9_10

Indications for Radiotherapy

Radiotherapy may be considered for all stages of KC of the extremity, especially when surgery is not recommended, or in the post-operative setting (for example, for positive or close margins) (Table 10.1).

In a large retrospective series from the United Kingdom [5], the authors reported on 541 primary KCs of the hand treated with surgery. Of these, 78% were cSCC, 11.3% were BCC and 3.9% were melanoma. There was a significant increased risk of regional lymph node metastases for web spaces or dorsum of the proximal phalanges as compared to other hand skin sites. The rate of regional lymph node metastases was 4.6% for web spaces or dorsum of the proximal phalanges compared to 1% for other hand areas ($p = 0.0275$). The superficial lymphatic plexus draining the digits and palmar surface converge on the dorsum of the hand. It has been hypothesized that malignancies originating on the thinner epidermis and dermis located in the dorsum of the hand have a greater propensity to invade and spread via these lymphatic channels.

The use of RT for hand sites has been published as a few case reports in the literature [6]. While there have been no direct comparisons between surgery and RT for hand sites, RT is generally considered in cases which are not amenable to curative surgery or when surgery is deemed to result in less favourable cosmetic or functional outcome.

Historically, there have been concerns regarding the use of RT for lower extremities, especially located below the knee, due to the risk of poor wound healing and risk of radiation necrosis [7, 8]. The risk of radiation injury to leg sites has been noted particularly in those with peripheral vascular disease, diabetes and smoking habit [9, 10]. Barnes and colleagues [8] reported on 39 below-the-knee skin sites in 25 patients treated with RT. With a mean follow-up time of 19 months, the crude complete response, partial response and progression rates were 65%, 19% and 16%, respectively. Seventeen percent of patients developed grade 3 skin toxicity. There was no grade 4 or 5 toxicity reported. The authors concluded that for below-the-knee skin cancer patients not eligible for surgery, RT is an option with a moderate chance of complete response (65%) and 17% risk of poor wound healing/radiation necrosis.

In the post-operative setting, adjuvant RT is given for close or positive margins. The use of post-operative RT for other high-risk features such as perineural invasion is controversial. A systematic review of surgery monotherapy versus surgery and adjuvant RT in high-risk cSCC [11] concluded that cure rates were high when surgical margins were clear. The current data suffers from small numbers making it insufficient to identify high-risk factors, which would make post-operative adjuvant

Table 10.1 Indications summary

Intent	Indications
Curative	Localized KC site +/− regional involved site (primary radiotherapy or post-operative, adjuvant)
Palliative	Tumour factors: locally advanced, metastatic Patient factors: frailty/functional status, comorbidities

radiation beneficial. Perineural invasion affecting larger nerves was associated with poorer prognosis.

Based on guidelines [12] and extrapolating from the head and neck literature, a therapeutic lymph node dissection should be performed in clinically or radiographically detected lymph node metastasis.

Regional nodal metastases may also be treated with RT in an adjuvant setting after surgery (for residual disease or for adverse features seen in the regional surgical specimen such as extracapsular extension and significant nodal burden). Radiotherapy may also be given as primary therapy for unresectable regional metastases.

For locally advanced, regionally advanced or metastatic KC, RT may be given with palliative/symptom control intent.

Radiotherapy Treatment Approach

Numerous RT techniques are available for treating extremity KC sites. These include:

1. Direct electrons
2. Direct orthovoltage
3. Parallel opposed photon fields
4. Intensity-modulated radiation therapy (IMRT) or volumetric modulated arc therapy (VMAT) preferred, for example, on convex or concave surfaces [13]
5. Surface mould brachytherapy
6. Interstitial brachytherapy

For non-orthovoltage external beam modalities, bolus is used to increase the skin surface dose. In addition, a strip of skin will be spared from radiation in case of large tumours to reduce the risk of post-radiotherapy lymphedema.

The best RT technique is chosen by the following considerations

1. Target coverage
2. Organs at risk dose minimization
3. Availability of the RT technique
4. Patient tolerance for radiation set-ups. For example, orthovoltage machines are capable of treating patients in the sitting position, whereas linac machines generally require that the patient be supine

Treatment Planning

The following RT volumes are delineated

1. Gross tumour volume (GTV): the visible, palpable tumour as identified on physical examination (which may include imaging)
2. Clinical target volume (CTV): the margin added to GTV to include microscopic spread (e.g. 1 cm)

3. Planning treatment volume (PTV): the margin added to CTV to include day-to-day variation and organ movement (e.g. 1 cm)

Figure 10.1 shows two leg nodules of basal cell skin cancer. The GTV is marked. A margin (2 cm total) is added for CTV and PTV. Penumbra (0.75 cm) is added to PTV to achieve dose to the field edge as marked in the outer circle.

Two oblique 6 MV photon fields with daily bolus (1 cm) were used (Fig. 10.2) to treat this volume to 50 Gy in 20 daily fractions:

VMAT plan can result in low-dose spillage over the healthy tissue and hence is not routinely recommended (Fig. 10.3a, b).

Fig. 10.1 Basal cell skin cancer of the leg

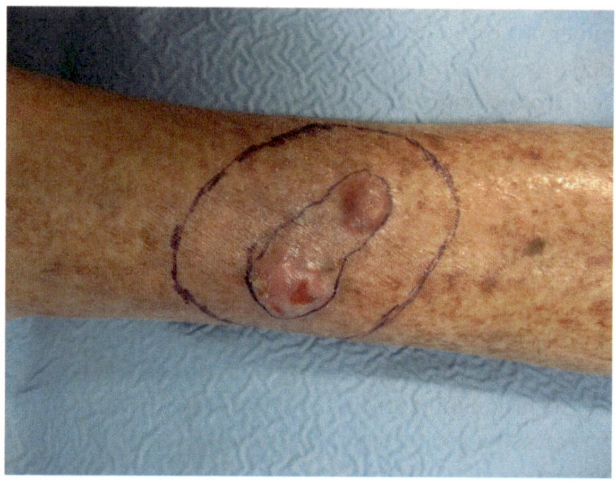

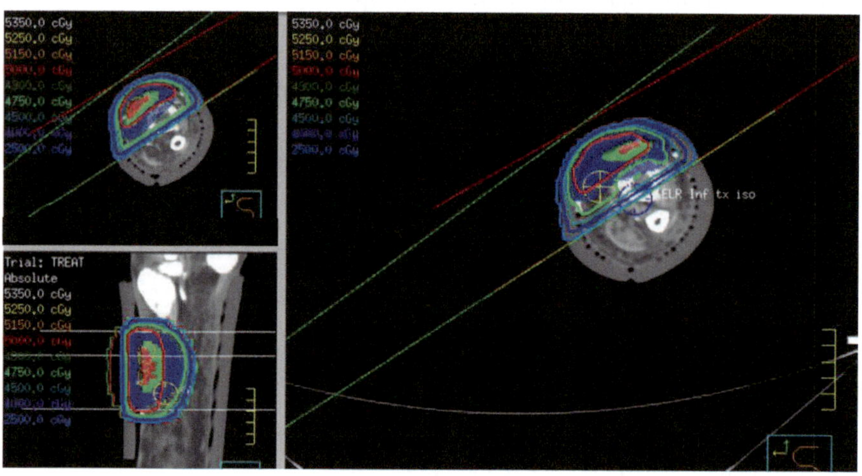

Fig. 10.2 Oblique 6 MV photon fields

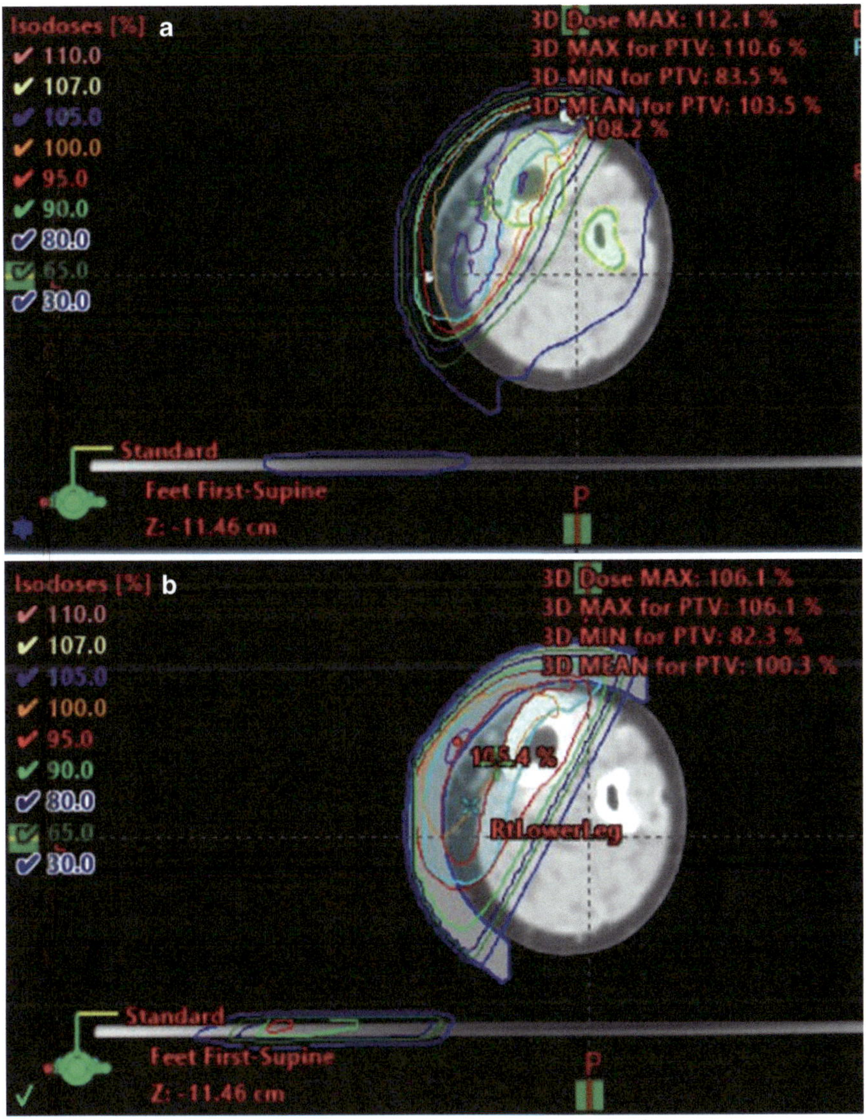

Fig. 10.3 Shows plans generated with VMAT (**a**) vs. 3D CRT (FiF IMRT) (**b**). VMAT causes significant low-dose spillage over normal tissue

Dose

Common radical dose fractionation schemes [14–23] are listed in Table 10.2. Caution is exercised when considering these radical dose fractionation schemes for below-the-knee sites due to risk of radiation necrosis particularly in patients with higher risk (e.g. patients with diabetes, vascular disease, smoking habit).

Table 10.2 Dose fractionation schemes

Hypofractionated regimens
35 Gy in 5 daily fractions over 5 days (or every other day) (tumour diameter <2 cm)
40–45 Gy in 10 daily fractions over 2 weeks
50 Gy in 15 daily fractions over 3 weeks
50–55 Gy in 20 daily fractions over 4 weeks
Conventionally fractionated regimens
60–66 Gy in 30–33 daily fractions over 6–6.5 weeks
64 Gy in 32 daily fractions over 6.2 weeks
Palliative dose fractionation examples
20 Gy in 5 daily fractions over 1 week
30 Gy in 10 daily fractions over 2 weeks
24 Gy in 3 daily fractions, each fraction given on days 0, 7 and 21

Treatment-Related Side Effects

Possible treatment-related side effects include acute skin reactions (redness, dry desquamation, moist desquamation). Late skin effects include skin pallor or hyperpigmentation, atrophy, telangiectasia, poor wound healing and radiation necrosis.

For regional lymph node RT, possible side effects include skin effects as listed above and also risk of lymphedema, brachial plexopathy for axillary sites, bowel toxicity and lymphedema for pelvic/inguinal lymph node sites.

Outcomes

For RT to lower extremities, one study included both radical intent radiation and palliative intent RT [8]. For these patients with below-the-knee sites treated with a variety of radiation schedules, the overall complete response rate was 65%. There is a lack of RT outcomes reported in the literature specifically examining extremity sites.

References

1. Stern RS. Prevalence of a history of skin cancer in 2007: results of an incidence-based model. Arch Dermatol. 2010;146(3):279–82.
2. Gallagher RP, Ma B, McLean DI, et al. Trends in basal cell carcinoma, squamous cell carcinoma and melanoma of the skin from 1973 through 1987. J Am Acad Dermatol. 1190;23(3, pt1):413–21.

3. Armstrong BK, Kricker A. The epidemiology of UV induced skin cancer. J Photochem Photobiol B. 2001;63(1–3):8–18.
4. Subramaniam P, Olsen CM, Thompson BS, et al. Anatomical distributions of basal cell carcinoma and squamous cell carcinoma in a population-based study in Queensland, Australia. JAMA Dermatol. 2017;153(2):175–82.
5. Maciburko SJ, Townley WA, Hollowood K, Giele HP. Skin cancers of the hand: a series of 541 malignancies. Plast Reconstr Surg. 2012;129(6):1329–36.
6. Brewer CF, Deutsch CJ, Jemec B. Is radiation therapy as primary treatment modality for squamous cell carcinoma of the hand the best choice? Case series and review of the literature. Dermatol Online J. 2020;26(6):13030/qt0mx961gq.
7. Dixon A. Managing skin cancer below the knee. Aust Fam Phys. 2006;35(10):785–6.
8. Barnes EA, Sinclair E, Assaad D, Fialkov J, Antonyshyn O, Tsao MN. Radiation for below the knee skin cancers: a single institution experience. J Dermatol Treat. 2020;31(6):563–6.
9. Clarke P. Nonmelanoma skin cancers - treatment options. Aust Fam Physician. 2012;41:476–80.
10. Feldmeier JJ, Heimbach RD, Davolt DA, et al. Hyperbaric oxygen in the treatment of delayed radiation injuries of the extremities. Undersea Hyperb Med. 2000;27:15–9.
11. Jambusaria-Pahlajani A, Miller CJ, Quon H, Smith N, Klein RQ, Schmults CD. Surgical monotherapy versus surgery plus adjuvant radiotherapy in high-risk cutaneous squamous cell carcinoma: a systematic review of outcomes. Dermatol Surg. 2009;35:574–85.
12. Stratigos AJ, Garbe C, Dessinioti C, European Dermatology Forum (EDF), the European Association of Dermato-Oncology (EADO) and the European Organization for Research and Treatment of Cancer (EORTC), et al. European interdisciplinary guideline on invasive squamous cell carcinoma of the skin: part 2. Treatment. Eur J Cancer. 2020;128:83–102.
13. Fitzgerald E, Miles W, Fenton P, et al. Intensity-modulated radiation therapy to bilateral lower limb extremities concurrently: a planning case study. J Med Radiat Sci. 2014;61(3):210–5.
14. Likhacheva A, Awan M, Barker CA, et al. Definitive and postoperative radiation therapy for basal and squamous cell cancers of the skin: executive summary of an American Society for Radiation Oncology clinical practice guideline. Pract Radiat Oncol. 2020;10(1):8–20.
15. Veness MJ, Delishaj D, Barnes EA, et al. Current role of radiotherapy in non-melanoma skin cancer statement of search strategies used and radiotherapy in non-melanoma skin cancer. Clin Oncol. 2019;31(11):749–58.
16. Keohane SG, Botting J, Budny PG, et al. British Association of Dermatologists guidelines for the management of people with cutaneous squamous carcinoma 2020. Br J Dermatol. 2021;184:384–5.
17. Nasr I, McGrath EJ, Harwood CA, et al. British Association of Dermatologists guidelines for the management of adults with basal cell carcinoma 2021. Br J Dermatol. 2021;185:899.
18. Veness MJ. Hypofractionated radiotherapy in patients with non-melanoma skin cancer in the post COVID-19 era: time to reconsider its role for most patients. J Med Imaging Radiat Oncol. 2020;64(4):591–4.
19. Thomson DJ, Yom SS, Saeed H, et al. Radiation fractionation schedules published during the COVID-19 pandemic: a systematic review of the quality of evidence and recommendations for future development. Int J Radiat Oncol Biol Phys. 2020;108(2):379–89.
20. Rembielak A, Sykes AJ, Fife K, et al. Radiotherapy and systemic treatment for non-melanoma skin cancer in the COVID-19 pandemic. Clin Oncol (R Coll Radiol). 2020;32(7):417–9.
21. National Comprehensive Cancer Network (NCCN) clinical practice guidelines in oncology. Basal cell skin cancer Version 1. 2020.
22. National Comprehensive Cancer Network (NCCN) clinical practice guidelines in oncology. Squamous cell skin cancer. Version 1. 2020.
23. McPartlin AJ, Slevin NJ, Sykes AJ, et al. Radiotherapy treatment of non-melanoma skin cancer: a survey of current UK practice and commentary. Br J Radiol. 2014;87:20140501.

Chapter 11
Primary Melanoma and Lentigo Maligna

Angela M. Hong

Melanoma is a malignant tumor of melanocytes. Melanoma accounts for 1.7% of global cancer diagnoses and is the fifth most common cancer in the USA [1]. However, mortality is decreasing owing mainly to the increased awareness, early detection, and advances in targeted and immunotherapies [2]. The clinical subtypes are:

- Superficial spreading (most common)
- Nodular
- Lentigo maligna
- Acral lentiginous (palmar/plantar and subuncal)
- Miscellaneous
  - Desmoplastic
  - Mucosal lentiginous (oral and genital)

The Cancer Genome Atlas (TCGA) Network has identified four major genomic subtypes of malignant melanoma [3]:

- BRAF mutant
- RAS mutant
- NF1 mutant
- Triple wild type

Targeted therapies and immunotherapies are effective treatments for melanoma and have significantly improved outcomes and are routinely used to treat high-risk and metastatic melanoma.

A. M. Hong (✉)
Melanoma Institute Australia, Faculty of Medicine and Health, University of Sydney, Sydney, NSW, Australia
e-mail: angela.hong@sydney.edu.au

K. J. Joseph et al. (eds.), *Radiotherapy in Skin Cancer*,
https://doi.org/10.1007/978-3-031-44316-9_11

Indications for Radiotherapy

Primary Melanoma

Wide local resection is the primary definitive treatment of cutaneous primary melanoma. Radiotherapy is indicated as an adjuvant treatment in selected cases with an aim to improve local control based on mostly retrospective data. The pathological features associated with higher risk of local recurrence that warrant consideration of adjuvant RT are microsatellitosis, desmoplasia, perineural invasion, and lymphovascular invasion. In cases where anatomic constraints may limit the ability to obtain widely negative margins, particularly in the head and neck, adjuvant RT has also been effectively used in the setting of either positive or close margins. Adjuvant RT may also be considered after excision of a local recurrence. In the uncommon scenario where the primary melanoma is not operable (e.g., inoperability because of medical comorbidities or proximity to vital structures such as the eye), definitive RT may be considered at the primary site. There are very limited data regarding the effectiveness of RT in this setting.

Desmoplastic Melanoma

Desmoplastic melanoma is an uncommon melanoma subtype that accounts for approximately 1–4% of all melanomas. The clinical behavior differs from that of non-desmoplastic melanoma [4–6]. Desmoplastic melanoma is frequently associated with perineural spread (neurotropism) and has been associated with an increased local failure rate. Occasionally, large named nerves can be involved, a clinical scenario that can be particularly troublesome to manage when there is tumor extension along cranial nerves and their branches from a cutaneous primary site on the head or neck towards the base of the skull [7].

There is no randomized trial defining the role of adjuvant RT after complete resection of desmoplastic melanoma with or without neurotropism. However, multiple case series support the use of adjuvant RT [4, 6–8]. The largest series, from the Melanoma Institute Australia, included 671 patients with neurotropic melanomas in which 72% were desmoplastic melanoma. In this study, adjuvant RT was associated with half the risk of local recurrence compared with surgery alone if microscopic margins were <8 mm. In another study of 277 patients where 113 patients received adjuvant RT, the overall 5-year local control rate for patients who received RT was significantly better compared with those who did not (86% vs. 46%, hazard ratio 0.15, 95% CI 0.06–0.39) [8]. For those with positive resection margins, the local recurrence rate was 14% vs. 54% ($P = 0.004$) in those who did not receive adjuvant RT. For those with negative margins, there was a trend towards improved local control with adjuvant RT (95% vs. 76%).

Despite the lack of randomized data, multiple national guidelines recommend that if excision margins are considered to be inadequate, adjuvant RT to the primary site is recommended for desmoplastic and neurotropic melanomas, for improvement in local control [9–14]. The American Academy of Dermatology guidelines recommend RT for patients with desmoplastic melanoma with narrow margins or high-risk features such as Breslow thickness >4 mm [13]. The Australian guidelines recommended RT for <8 mm pathological margin [9], and the German guidelines recommended RT for <1 cm margin [10]. The South African guidelines recommend adjuvant RT be used for those with recurrent desmoplastic or neurotropic melanomas [15].

In summary, RT to the primary site may be indicated for primary melanoma with perineural spread. In addition, RT should be considered in desmoplastic melanoma that has not been resected with wide margins.

Lentigo Maligna

Lentigo maligna (LM) is a form of melanoma in situ that generally occurs on exposed sun-damaged skin of elderly people. It has a slow growth rate and low potential to develop into invasive disease. There is currently no randomized data comparing the efficacy of the three main treatment modalities (surgery, RT, topical imiquimod) for LM. The results from a prospective randomized phase 3 trial comparing RT with topical imiquimod in LM will be reported in late 2023 (ClinicalTrials.gov Identifier: NCT02394132). Consensus-based international guidelines recommend surgery as a primary treatment for LM, allowing a pathologic assessment of invasion and margins. For large area of LM in cosmetically sensitive areas of the face or when performing a wide excision is difficult, nonsurgical treatments can be considered. Definitive RT with superficial energy radiation is a feasible alternative option and is a recommended nonsurgical option by several national guidelines [16, 17]. The response to RT is typically slow with response assessment at least 6 months after completion, unless there is clear sign of disease progression or concern of development of invasion.

In a large series of 593 patients with LM and early LM melanoma treated with superficial energy RT (RT alone, $n = 350$; partial excision followed by RT, $n = 71$; radical excision followed by adjuvant RT, $n = 172$), the complete clearance rates were 83%, 90%, and 97%, respectively [18]. A recent systematic review of 14 retrospective studies of 1075 LM cases reported that local recurrence rates ranged from 0 to 31% [19]. The reported cosmetic outcomes were good to excellent in the majority of the studies. Due to retrospective nature of the studies, there were variations in follow-up time, definition of local control, and assessment of cosmetic outcome. A wide range of dose fractionation and techniques have been used in these studies.

Treatment Planning

Target Volume

For desmoplastic neurotropic melanoma, the surgical bed (defined as the volume of tissue incorporating the excisional scar superficially excluding scar from any local flap) and any visible cavity on CT scan (including deep tissues down to the next uninvolved tissue layer, e.g., muscle, bone, fat) should be defined on CT scan. The clinical target volume (CTV) is an additional 1.5 cm margin in all directions, adjusted so that anatomical boundaries are respected, e.g., skin surface and bone margin. A planning target volume (PTV) of 0.5–1 cm is then given depending on tumor location and immobilization used to treat the lesion.

For LM treatment with superficial/orthovoltage RT, the treatment field is defined as the clinical disease or area defined by confocal microscopy with a 10 mm margin (clinical markup) if possible, depending on anatomical constraints (Fig. 11.1).

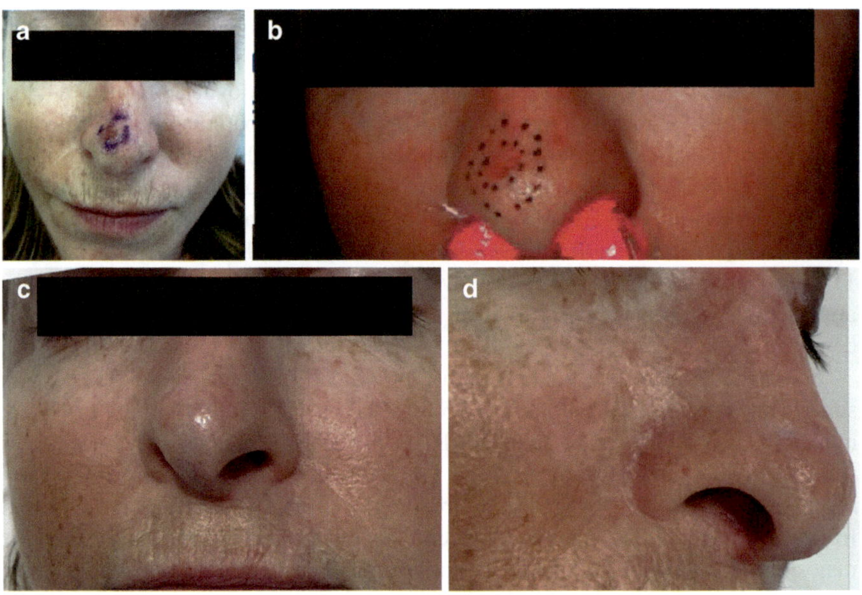

Fig. 11.1 (**a**) 60-Year-old lady with a lentigo maligna on the nose. Patient declined wide local excision with a skin graft repair and received superficial RT. The extent of the disease was defined by reflectance confocal microscopy as marked. (**b**) The treatment field was 10 mm around the extent of the disease. The area was treated to 56 Gy in 28 fractions using 100 kVp. (**c**, **d**) Complete response and excellent cosmetic result 24 months post-RT

Dose Fractionation

Desmoplastic Melanoma

The optimal dose fractionation for adjuvant RT has not been established. It can be tailored to the location, treatment volume and patient comorbidity, and travel distance to the treatment center. Suggested dose schedules in the setting of negative margins are 48–56 Gy in 20–28 daily fractions or hypofractionated regimens such as 30 Gy in 5 fractions (twice a week). For positive margins or where further excision is not recommended, higher dose equivalent of 60–66 Gy in 30–33 fractions should be considered.

Lentigo Maligna

The recommended definitive dose is at least 56 Gy in 28 daily fractions or equivalent, and adjuvant dose should be 50 Gy in 2–2.5 Gy fractions or equivalent using superficial/orthovoltage RT to ensure the adequate coverage of the skin appendage to a depth of about 4.5–5 mm.

Palliative Radiotherapy

Palliative RT can be given for local recurrence and skin metastasis. Local recurrence, in-transit disease, or soft tissue metastasis can cause significant local symptoms such as pain, fungation, compression of surrounding normal structures, or bleeding. Palliative RT can provide symptomatic benefit and prolonged local disease control. The dose fractionation will depend on the size, location, and extent of disease elsewhere. A range of suitable schedules are 8 Gy in 1 fraction, 20 Gy in 5 daily fractions, 30 Gy in 10 daily fractions, and 30 Gy in 5 fractions (twice a week) (Fig. 11.2). Dose escalation with stereotactic body (SBRT) techniques, especially for brain and spinal metastases, can be considered.

Treatment-Related Side Effects

The RT is generally well tolerated apart from acute toxicity such as fatigue, and local effects (skin erythema, desquamation) depend on tumor location. Treatment in the head and neck region may cause temporary mucositis. Potential long-term effects are alopecia within treatment area, pigmentation, and fibrosis and depend on the dose delivered.

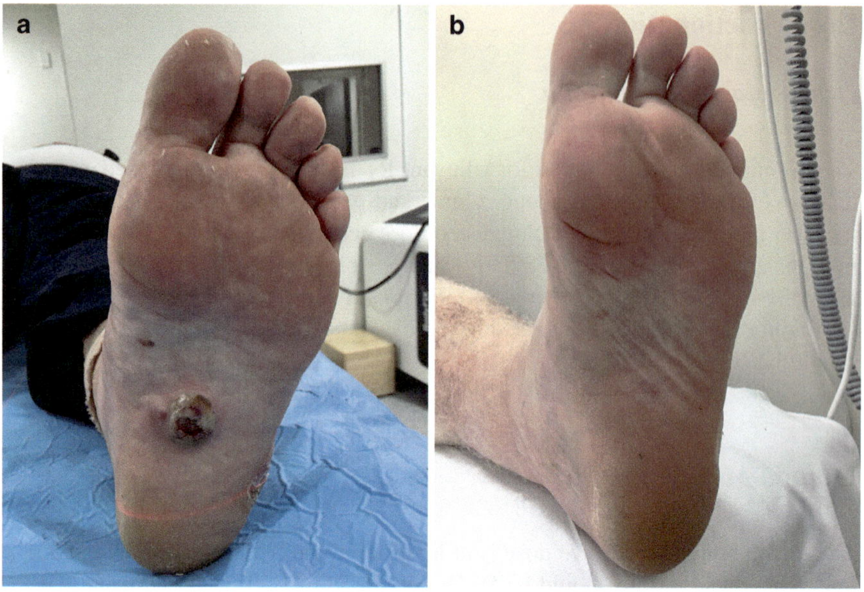

Fig. 11.2 (**a**) 55-Year-old man with a fungating soft tissue deposit of metastatic melanoma on the sole of his left foot. (**b**) Complete response 3 months after 30 Gy in 10 fractions of radiotherapy

References

1. Ferlay J, Ervik M, Lam F, Colombet M, Mery L, Piñeros M, et al. Global cancer observatory: cancer today. International Agency for Research on Cancer. 2023. https://gco.iarc.fr/today/home.
2. Siegel RL, Miller KD, Fuchs HE, Jemal A. Cancer statistics, 2022. CA Cancer J Clin. 2022;72(1):7–33.
3. Cancer Genome Atlas Network. Genomic classification of cutaneous melanoma. Cell. 2015;161(7):1681–96.
4. Chen JY, Hruby G, Scolyer RA, Murali R, Hong A, FitzGerald P, et al. Desmoplastic neurotropic melanoma: a clinicopathologic analysis of 128 cases. Cancer. 2008;113(10):2770–8.
5. Scolyer RA, Thompson JF. Desmoplastic melanoma: a heterogeneous entity in which subclassification as "pure" or "mixed" may have important prognostic significance. Ann Surg Oncol. 2005;12(3):197–9.
6. Varey AHR, Goumas C, Hong AM, Mann GJ, Fogarty GB, Stretch JR, et al. Neurotropic melanoma: an analysis of the clinicopathological features, management strategies and survival outcomes for 671 patients treated at a tertiary referral center. Mod Pathol. 2017;30(11):1538–50.
7. Guadagnolo BA, Prieto V, Weber R, Ross MI, Zagars GK. The role of adjuvant radiotherapy in the local management of desmoplastic melanoma. Cancer. 2014;120(9):1361–8.
8. Strom T, Caudell JJ, Han D, Zager JS, Yu D, Cruse CW, et al. Radiotherapy influences local control in patients with desmoplastic melanoma. Cancer. 2014;120(9):1369–78.
9. Hughes TM, Gyorki D, Kelly J, Stretch J, Scolyer RA, Varey A, et al. Primary desmoplastic and neurotropic melanomas Australia. Cancer Council Australia. 2018. https://wiki.cancer.org.au/australiawiki/index.php?oldid=187679.
10. Arbeitsgemeinschaft der Wissenschaftlichen Medizinischen Fachgesellschaften e.V. (AWMF). S3-Leitlinie zur Diagnostik, Therapie und Nachsorge des Melanoms: Arbeitsgemeinschaft

der Wissenschaftlichen Medizinischen Fachgesellschaften e.V. (AWMF). 2019. https://www.leitlinienprogramm-onkologie.de/fileadmin/user_upload/Downloads/Leitlinien/Melanom/Melanom_Version_3/LL_Melanom_Langversion_3.2.pdf.

11. Coit DG, Thompson JA, Albertini MR, Barker C, Carson WE III, Contreras C, et al. Cutaneous melanoma, version 2.2019, NCCN Clinical Practice Guidelines in Oncology. J Natl Compr Cancer Netw. 2019;17(4):e1.
12. Berrocal A, Arance A, Castellon V, de la Cruz L, Espinosa E, Cao MG, et al. SEOM clinical guideline for the management of malignant melanoma (2017). Clin Trans Oncol. 2018;20(1):69–74.
13. Swetter SM, Tsao H, Bichakjian CK, Curiel-Lewandrowski C, Elder DE, Gershenwald JE, et al. Guidelines of care for the management of primary cutaneous melanoma. J Am Acad Dermatol. 2019;80(1):208–50.
14. Rutkowski P, Wysocki PJ, Nasierowska-Guttmejer A, Fijuth J, Kalinka-Warzocha E, Świtaj T, et al. Cutaneous melanoma—diagnostic and therapeutic guidelines in 2016. Oncol Clin Pract. 2015;11(4):216–331.
15. Whitaker D, Sinclair W. Melanoma advisory board—guideline on the management of melanoma. J S Afr Med. 2004;94(8):699–707.
16. Garbe C, Amaral T, Peris K, Hauschild A, Arenberger P, Basset-Seguin N, et al. European consensus-based interdisciplinary guideline for melanoma. Part 2: treatment—update 2022. Eur J Cancer. 2022;170:256–84.
17. Robinson M, Primiero C, Guitera P, Hong A, Scolyer RA, Stretch JR, et al. Evidence-based clinical practice guidelines for the management of patients with lentigo maligna. Dermatology. 2020;236(2):111–6.
18. Hedblad MA, Mallbris L. Grenz ray treatment of lentigo maligna and early lentigo maligna melanoma. J Am Acad Dermatol. 2012;67(1):60–8.
19. Hendrickx A, Cozzio A, Plasswilm L, Panje CM. Radiotherapy for lentigo maligna and lentigo maligna melanoma—a systematic review. Radiat Oncol. 2020;15(1):174.

Chapter 12
Merkel Cell Carcinoma

Michael. J. Veness

Merkel cell carcinoma (MCC) is a rare skin cancer with median age at diagnosis between 70 and 75 years old and involving the head and neck in 40–50% of cases. Chronic ultraviolet exposure and immunosuppression are risk factors. MCC is associated with a highly prevalent virus, the Merkel cell polyomavirus (MCPyV) although the prevalence varies in distinct populations [1]. MCC is notoriously difficult to diagnose on clinical grounds, and lesions tend to be reddish/violaceous in appearance and are often non-ulcerative, nodular and progress rapidly [2] (Fig. 12.1a).

Histopathology is of small monomorphous round cells with scanty cytoplasm that belong to the family of "small round bell cell tumours". Most stain positive for the neuroendocrine marker cytokeratin 20 (CK 20) often in a perinuclear dot-like distribution and are negative for cytokeratin 7 (CK 7) and thyroid transcription factor 1 (TTF-1) [1]. Other neuroendocrine markers such as chromogranin A and synaptophysin are usually positive.

Extent (or stage) of disease (local vs. locoregional) is highly prognostic [3]. The extent of nodal disease (microscopic vs. macroscopic) is also prognostic. It is important to establish the extent of a patient's MCC at diagnosis as this will impact both management and prognosis. With most (50–60%) patients presenting with a primary lesion (stage I/II), there is a need to investigate draining lymph nodes (so-called sentinel nodes) as the incidence of subclinical spread is high (30–50%). Clinical examination alone will not detect subclinically involved nodes, and there is a need for investigations. Sentinel lymph node biopsy (SLNB) is recommended in

M. J. Veness (✉)
Department of Radiation Oncology, Crown Princess Mary Cancer Centre, Westmead Hospital, Sydney, NSW, Australia

University of Sydney, Sydney, NSW, Australia
e-mail: michael.veness@health.nsw.gov.au

K. J. Joseph et al. (eds.), *Radiotherapy in Skin Cancer*,
https://doi.org/10.1007/978-3-031-44316-9_12

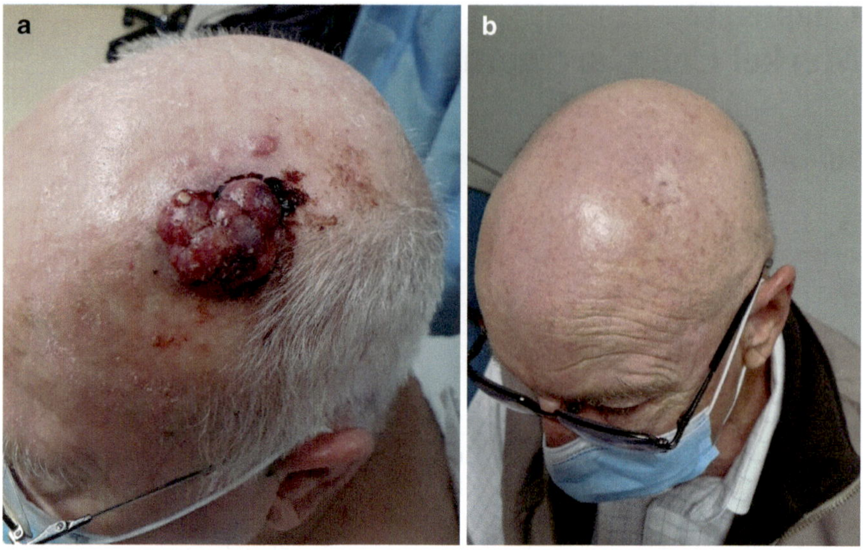

Fig. 12.1 (**a**) 72-Year-old male with a rapidly progressing left scalp MCC. Note the expansile appearance and nearby satellite lesions. The patient was treated with definitive RT including elective treatment of his ipsilateral parotid and upper neck lymph nodes. (**b**) He received 55 Gy in 25 fractions to his left hemi-scalp using VMAT and the addition of bolus and 50 Gy in 25 fractions to his parotid and upper cervical nodes and achieved complete clinical response shortly after completing his RT

clinically node-negative patients [4]. Radiotherapy (RT) plays an essential role in the management of patients with MCC [5].

Indications for Radiotherapy

Adjuvant (Primary Site)

The indications for adjuvant local RT to the primary site lack high-level evidence but will improve local control and should be recommended in most patients [6]. There is no consensus on whether there is a treatment benefit based on tumour size or margin status. RT to the primary site may be omitted for patients with no underlying high-risk factors such as immunosuppression, and if the primary tumour is small (<1 cm), excised with wide margins (1–2 cm), and pathology shows no lymphovascular invasion or a positive SLNB. These so-called favourable patients are uncommon. When margins are close (<1 cm), or positive, and re-excision is not feasible, patients should always be offered adjuvant RT to decrease the risk of local recurrence.

Adjuvant (Regional)

Following regional surgery, or a positive SLNB, patients should be recommended adjuvant regional RT. If feasible, the primary site (if present), in-transit tissue and involved regional RT should be encompassed in one treatment volume (or field), but usually this is only possible for head and neck-located lesions, e.g. treating temple MCC and draining parotid gland nodes including in-transit tissue.

Definitive

In many patients, the extent of disease (local or regional) at presentation is technically or medically inoperable, or occasionally patients decline surgery. Up to 10–15% of patients present with MCC involving a lymph node but without an identifiable primary (or index) lesion. These patients should be considered for a nonsurgical approach utilising definitive RT [7] (Fig. 12.2a, b). Few patients undergoing regional surgery will avoid the need for adjuvant regional RT in any case. It is recommended that not only the involved nodes be irradiated but also elective RT to nearby uninvolved nodes. For example, definitive RT to a parotid gland metastatic node should also electively include the next echelon upper cervical neck nodes.

Palliative

Patients of poor performance status should be considered for a lower dose hypofractionation schedule, which can still achieve excellent tumour regression. Treatment should be limited to gross disease only and not electively treat nodes (Fig. 12.3).

Treatment Approach

Depending on disease location, size and thickness, occasionally relatively small fields on flat surfaces may be treated with superficial/orthovoltage energy photons or alternatively low/moderate-energy electrons (6–9 MeV) with the addition of tissue equivalent bolus. This approach is more often utilised in the palliative setting and has limitations in treating wider fields (or volumes) that may include in-transit and/or regional RT.

The majority of patients are better treated with megavoltage 3-dimensional conformal RT (3D-CRT) or highly conformal intensity-modulated RT (IMRT) or volumetric arc therapy (VMAT), and it is often the optimal approach that also allows for the delivery of a sequential integrated boost (SIB). There are very few scenarios

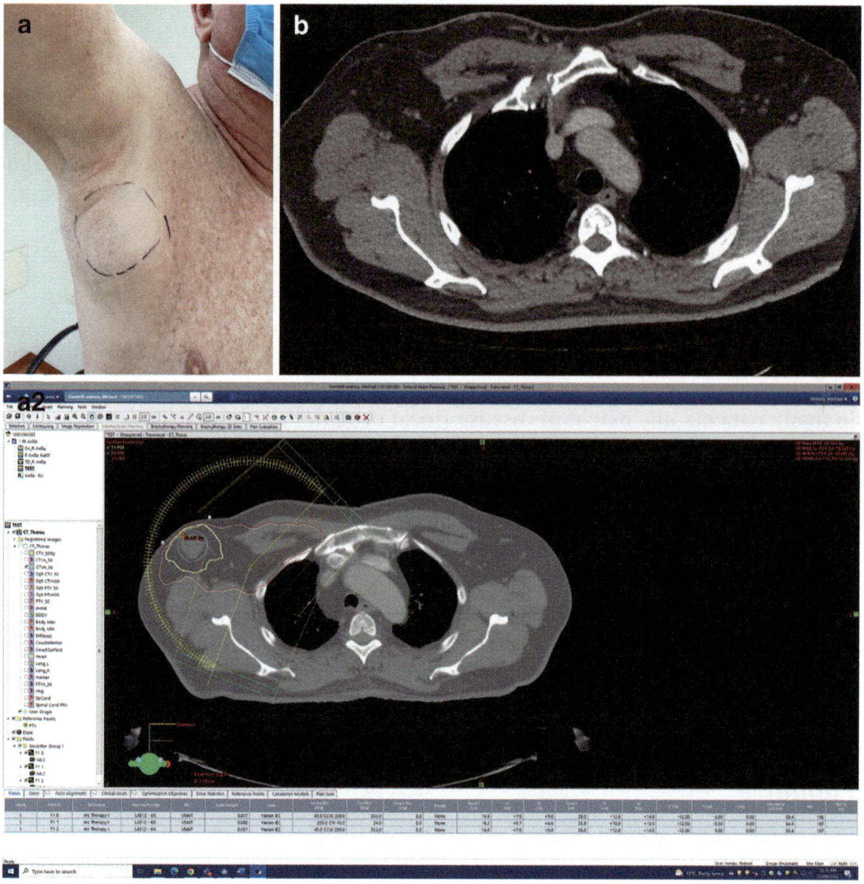

Fig. 12.2 (**a**) 66-Year-old male with a 5 cm right-side axillary node of unknown primary origin. He was treated with VMAT to a dose of 55 Gy in 25 fractions to the involved node and 50 Gy to nearby uninvolved nodal levels. He experienced complete clinical regression but relapsed 9 months later within mediastinal and para-aortic nodes. (**b**) 3 Months post-RT, he experienced complete clinical and metabolic (PET) response to treatment but shortly after developed distant para-aortic nodal relapse. He was commenced on immunotherapy after this relapse

whereby the advantages of accurately delivered IMRT/VMAT are outweighed by any disadvantages compared with an alternative approach. Sites such as the scalp or extremities or the requirement to treat a nodal region benefits from a conformal approach.

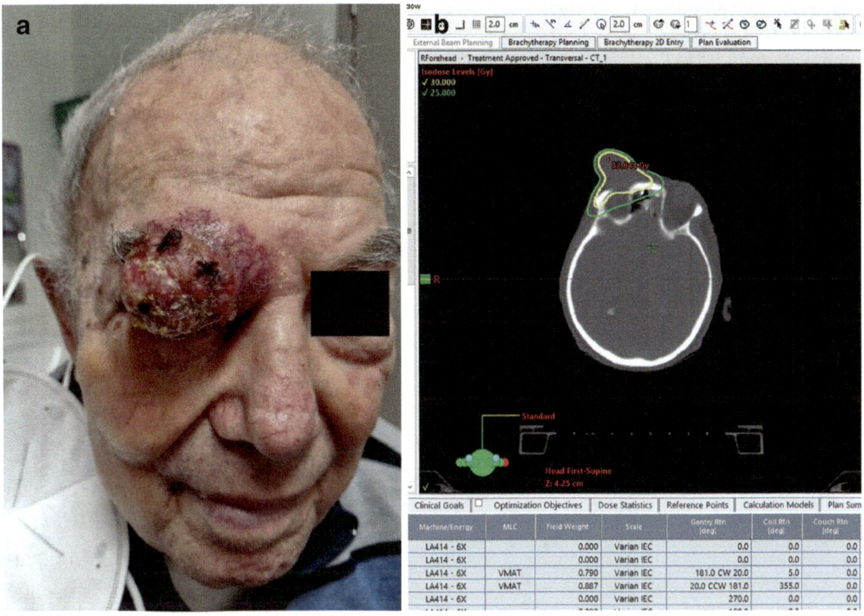

Fig. 12.3 (**a**) 88-Year-old male with a large rapidly enlarging right lower forehead MCC. He was of poor performance status and was treated with local palliative RT using VMAT to a dose of 30 Gy in 6 fractions twice per week. (**b**) Plan for patient highlighted in this figure. A GTV was delineated and a 5 mm expansion applied to achieve a PTV (no CTV). Bolus was not applied because of patient intolerance to this. The underlying anterior right orbit could not be spared without risking underdosing of the disease

Treatment Planning

Target Volume

Local Treatment

It is important that the prescribed dose is delivered to the skin surface as well as at depth. Bolus (0.5–1 cm) is required if using megavoltage photons or electrons. Accepting anatomical barriers such as bone or cartilage, patients should be treated with at least 3–5 cm margins especially peripherally beyond a lesion (GTV) or surgical bed (Fig. 12.4). The clinical target volume (CTV) can be reduced when critical organs at risk (OAR) are nearby. CTV at depth should be down to the fascial plan or periosteum of bone. Planning target volume (PTV) expansions of 3–5 mm are recommended. If clinicians utilise electrons, wider field margins are required and the dose is prescribed to 90% isodose line. Patients with lesions in close proximity to the eye may require an internal eye shield (if possible) inserted to protect the globe, and in these cases, superficial energy photons offer an advantage over electrons where thin (2–3 mm) lead shields may not be appropriate.

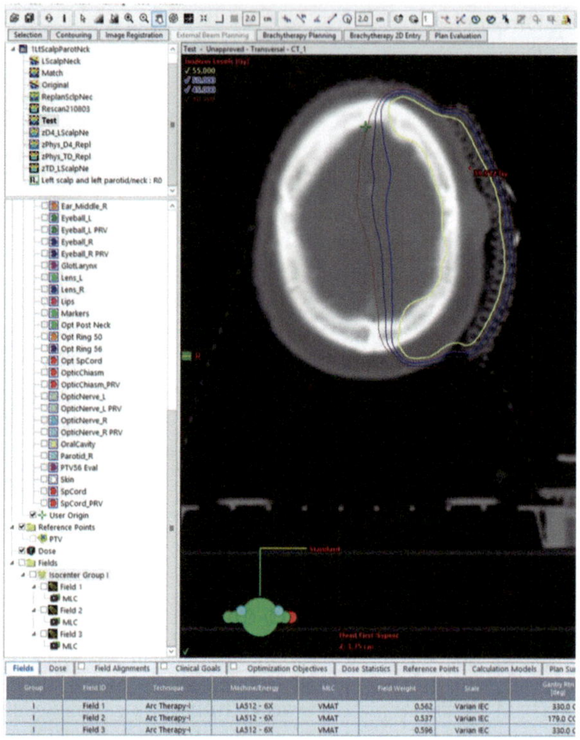

Fig. 12.4 Left-scalp MCC (see Fig. 12.1a) treated with wide-field VMAT with the addition of overlying bolus (1 cm). Note the extent of the CTV (4 cm) beyond the primary tumour as reflected in the 55 Gy isodose but cropped at the skull

Regional Treatment

Regional RT should be delivered with IMRT or VMAT allowing for the use of two dose levels delivering an SIB. Patients should have any diagnostic scans fused with the planning of CT. The administration of IV contrast should also be considered. Involved nodes are contoured and expanded 0.5–1 cm to achieve a CTV and 3–5 mm for a PTV. Elective lower dose RT should include the entire nodal region, e.g. remaining uninvolved neck, groin or axilla.

Palliative

Patients recommended palliative intent RT should have limited expansions applied to any GTV (primary or lymph node) so as to limit toxicity, especially in the head and neck (Fig. 12.3). GTV-to-CTV expansion should be limited to 5–10 mm and 3–5 mm CTV to PTV. Clinicians may decide not to generate a CTV. Wider expansions may be considered in non-critical sites or if subclinical disease is suspected. However, elective treatment beyond clinical or suspected clinical spread is usually not recommended.

Dose

MCC can be considered more responsive to RT compared with other more common skin cancers such as squamous and basal cell carcinoma. Clinical response in the setting of definitive and palliative settings can occur rapidly and often during treatment. Initiation of RT should be made a priority as MCC can rapidly progress (definitive RT) or recur shortly after surgery (adjuvant RT).

Adjuvant

The optimal adjuvant RT dose is unclear with doses of 50–60 Gy recommended. Noting the radiosensitivity of MCC, most patients are adequately treated with 50–55 Gy in 1.8–2 Gy daily fractions. Patients do not benefit from adjuvant doses of >60 Gy often prescribed in other cutaneous malignancies. A recent study suggested that patients treated with hypofractionation regimens in both the definitive and adjuvant settings, using >2 Gy fractions (45–50 Gy in 15–20 fractions and 30–35 Gy in 8–10 fractions), had a similar outcome compared to patients treated with 2 Gy fractions (50–60 Gy) [8]. These shorter hypofractionated RT regimens are likely to be effective in poor performance patients and should be considered as a more tolerable alternative to 4–5 weeks of weekday RT. One small series ($n = 12$) has suggested that a single fraction of 8 Gy is effective in the adjuvant setting in select patients that may not be suitable for multiple fractions of RT [9]. Lesions located on the lower limb because of the risk of poor wound healing and wound breakdown should not be prescribed doses >50–55 Gy.

Definitive

The unique radioresponsiveness of MCC provides the option of RT alone with doses in the range of 55–60 Gy achieving excellent in-field control (80–90%), even in the setting of large primary lesions and/or nodal metastasis [10]. In a systematic review of the literature, the authors documented an almost 90% in-field control rate following definitive RT with a mean dose delivered of just under 50 Gy [11]. Elective treatment to nearby uninvolved nodes may be delivered to a lower total dose (45–50 Gy).

Palliative

Hypofractionation is effective in older poor performance patients unable to tolerate longer schedules and can achieve excellent palliation (e.g. single 8–10 Gy fraction, 20 Gy in 5 fractions or 30 Gy in 10 fractions). At least one study has documented 45% complete response using an 8 Gy single fraction (including large tumours up to 16 cm) and almost 80% in-field lesion control [12].

Treatment-Related Side Effects

Treatment-related side effects are dependent on the site undergoing RT and the irradiated volume. Patients undergoing locoregional RT to the head and neck may experience oral cavity/oropharyngeal associated side effects such as xerostomia, loss of taste and odynophagia. Cutaneous reactions such as erythema and moist desquamation are to be expected but resolve within 2–3 weeks of completing treatment. Shorter hypofractionated courses are likely to be associated with less toxicity.

Outcomes

Many published series document a cause-specific mortality of 30–40% highlighting the poor outcome of many patients diagnosed with MCC. Death is usually a consequence of patients developing disseminated relapse while maintaining in-field locoregional control. Patients presenting with primary only disease have the best chance of cure. However, the outcome of patients can be unpredictable, and even patients with early-stage node-negative MCC can relapse and die while patients with advanced locoregional MCC may be cured. As a rule, it is unusual for patients to present with distant metastases, as opposed to the relapse setting, but patients with clinical nodal metastases should be considered at the most risk of doing so following treatment. The survival depends on the stage at diagnosis (5-year survival of 60–65% in stage I, 35–55% in stage II, 30–40% in stage III and ~10% in stage IV) [13].

Follow-Up

There is no consensus on an optimal follow-up regimen and appropriate investigations. Approximately 40% of patients will develop relapse, and as most (90%) that do so relapse within the first 2–3 years, it is advisable to schedule regular 2–3-monthly clinical reviews within this time frame. Following this, patients can be reviewed every 3–4 months with most discharged from follow-up after 5 years and considered cured.

The role of regular surveillance investigations in a clinically disease-free patient is unclear. Patients treated with definitive RT may be considered for a follow-up PET scan at 3–4 months posttreatment to establish if complete metabolic response has been achieved. Similarly, immunosuppressed patients may be considered for more frequent posttreatment investigations, although evidence to support this in improving outcome is lacking. The early detection of asymptomatic distant relapse may prompt the initiation of immunotherapy [14] and consequently regular 6-monthly whole-body CT scans may be warranted within the first 2–3 years.

References

1. Gauci M, Aristei C, Becker JC, et al. Diagnosis and treatment of Merkel cell carcinoma: European consensus-based interdisciplinary guideline—update 2022. Eur J Cancer. 2022;171:203–31.
2. Heath M, Jaimes N, Lemos B, et al. Clinical characteristics of Merkel cell carcinoma at diagnosis in 195 patients: the AEIOU features. J Am Acad Dermatol. 2008;58:375–81.
3. Joseph K, Wong J, Abraham A, et al. Patterns and predictors of relapse in Merkel cell carcinoma: results from a population-based study. Radiother Oncol. 2022;166:110–7.
4. Gunaratne DA, Howle JR, Veness MJ. Sentinel lymph node biopsy in Merkel cell carcinoma: a 15 year institutional experience and statistical analysis of 721 reported cases. Br J Dermatol. 2016;174:273–81.
5. Veness MJ. Radiation therapy in Merkel cell carcinoma. In: Wenz F, editor. Radiation oncology. Cham: Springer International Publishing AG, part of Springer Nature; 2018. https://doi.org/10.1007/978-3-319-52619-5_16-1.
6. Seesha R, Takagishi BS, Tessa E, et al. Postoperative radiation therapy is associated with a reduced risk of local recurrence among low risk Merkel cell carcinomas of the head and neck. Adv Radiat Oncol. 2016;1:244–51.
7. Foote M, Veness M, Zarate D, Poulsen M. Merkel cell carcinoma: the prognostic implications of an occult primary in stage IIIB (nodal) disease. J Am Acad Dermatol. 2012;67:395–9.
8. Liu K, Milligan M, Schoenfeld J, et al. Characterisation of clinical outcomes after shorter course hypofractionated and standard-course radiotherapy for stage I–III curatively treated Merkel cell carcinoma. Radio Oncol. 2022;173:32–40.
9. Cook M, Schaub S, Goof P, et al. Postoperative, single fraction radiation therapy in Merkel cell carcinoma of the head and neck. Adv Radiat Oncol. 2020;5:12481254.
10. Veness M, Howle J. Radiotherapy alone in patients with Merkel cell carcinoma: the Westmead hospital experience of 41 patients. Australas J Dermatol. 2015;56:19–24.
11. Gunaratne D, Howle J, Veness MJ. Definitive radiotherapy for Merkel cell carcinoma confers clinically meaningful in-field locoregional control: a review and analysis of the literature. J Am Acad Dermatol. 2017;77:142–48.e1.
12. Iyer J, Parvathanen U, Gooley T, et al. Single-fraction radiation therapy in patients with metastatic Merkel cell carcinoma. Cancer Med. 2015;4:1161–70.
13. Harms K, Healy M, Nghiem P, et al. Analysis of prognostic factors from 9387 Merkel cell carcinoma cases forms the basis for the new 8th edition AJCC staging system. Ann Surg Oncol. 2016;23:3564–71.
14. Hasmat S, Howle JR, Karikios DJ, Carlino MS, Veness MJ. Immunotherapy in advanced Merkel cell carcinoma: Sydney west cancer network experience. J Med Imaging Radiat Oncol. 2021;65:760–7.

Chapter 13
Primary Cutaneous Lymphomas

Karen Pat-Ming Chu

Introduction

Classification

Primary cutaneous lymphomas (PCLs) are a group of lymphomas that exhibit no signs of extracutaneous disease at diagnosis. The World Health Organization (WHO) and the European Organization for Research and Treatment of Cancer (EORTC) classification divides PCLs into primary cutaneous B cell lymphomas (PCBCLs) and primary cutaneous T cell lymphomas (PCTCLs). The vast majority of these cutaneous lymphomas are PCTCL (75%). Compared to prior classification systems, the WHO–EORTC classification takes into consideration the distinct immunophenotype, clinical behavior, and often superior outcomes of these PCLs compared to their nodal counterparts.

Epidemiology

The incidence of both types of cutaneous lymphomas has been rising based on the Surveillance, Epidemiology, and End Results (SEER) registry data [1]. A recent report indicates that the incidence of PCTCL has risen 0.61% per year between

K. P.-M. Chu (✉)
Department of Oncology, University of Alberta, Edmonton, AB, Canada

Division of Radiation Oncology, Cross Cancer Institute, Edmonton, AB, Canada
e-mail: Karen.Chu@albertahealthservices.ca

K. J. Joseph et al. (eds.), *Radiotherapy in Skin Cancer*,
https://doi.org/10.1007/978-3-031-44316-9_13

Table 13.1 Frequency and survival of common primary cutaneous lymphomas

WHO–EORTC classification	Frequency (%)	5-Year disease-specific survival (%)
PCTCL		
Mycosis fungoides	39	88
Folliculotropic mycosis fungoides	5	75
Sezary syndrome	2	36
Primary cutaneous CD30+ lymphoproliferative disorders	25	>95
Primary cutaneous CD4+ small/medium T cell lymphoproliferative disorder	6[a]	100
Primary cutaneous peripheral T cell lymphoma NOS	2	15
PCBCL		
Primary cutaneous marginal zone lymphoma	9	99
Primary cutaneous follicular lymphoma	12	95
Primary cutaneous diffuse large B cell lymphoma, leg type	4	56

Adapted from the WHO–EORTC classification (Willemze 2019)

[a]The frequency of primary cutaneous CD4+ small/medium T cell lymphoproliferative disorder may be underreported [3]

2000 and 2018. While the incidence of PCTCL is highest among men and African Americans, the incidence of PCBCL is highest among males and non-Hispanic whites [2]. In both types, diagnosis is most common in adults >50 years of age. While there are a wide variety of cutaneous lymphomas, mycosis fungoides (MF) represents the most common T cell lymphoma, and the most common cutaneous B cell lymphoma is represented by primary cutaneous follicular lymphoma (PCFL) (Table 13.1). However, it is important to note that the incidence of PCLs can vary in different parts of the world. One prime example is in Southeast Asian countries where MF is less common than other PCTCL. PCLs are rare entities that should be diagnosed and managed by a multidisciplinary team involving both oncology and dermatology.

Workup

Evaluation of PCLs requires a complete physical examination of the skin and lymph nodes. Organomegaly should be ruled out. Pathologic confirmation of lymphoma by core/excisional biopsy is required in addition to histology, cytogenetics, and immunophenotyping. Complete blood count with manual differentiation, chemistries, liver function tests, and lactate dehydrogenase can be used in conjunction with computer tomography imaging to rule out systemic involvement.

Primary Cutaneous T Cell Lymphoma

Staging of PCTCL is classified using a TNMB system of skin (T), nodal (N), and visceral (M) involvement. B refers to the involvement of Sezary cells in the blood. In patients with early MF where only patches or plaques are identified, skin-directed therapy is ideal. This can range from topical steroids to UV-based therapy to topical cytostatic therapy such as carmustine [4–6].

Indications for Radiotherapy

Radiotherapy (RT) is very effective in treating early MF for localized control. Disease limited to patches and plaques without extra-cutaneous involvement can be controlled with orthovoltage energy photons or electron therapy. Orthovoltage is often ideal given the sharp falloff of dose, thereby minimizing normal tissue toxicity. Further, given the propensity of recurrent skin lesions in PCTCL patients, minimizing the amount of skin irradiated with each course of treatment allows for easier planning and safer re-treatment if the patient presents with new MF lesions. Intensity-modulated radiation therapy (IMRT) and volumetric modulated arc therapy (VMAT) with bolus are also radiation technique options for skin targets not well suited for single-beam orthovoltage or electrons (e.g., due to deeply invasive tumors, significant irregular surface contour, proximity to organs at risk).

Treatment Planning

Target Volume

In these cases, the gross tumor volume (GTV) is comprised of the gross tumor visualized and palpated on physical examination or visible on imaging. Wires can be used for localization on CT simulation, and if available, pretreatment imaging can be fused with the CT simulation to ensure complete inclusion of the GTV. The clinical target volume (CTV) encompasses the GTV with an additional margin for microscopic spread, while anatomical boundaries not involved with microscopic cancer are excluded. Finally, a planning target volume (PTV) is applied to account for setup error or patient motion during treatment. The PTV is also dependent on the immobilization technique and may range from 0.5 cm in an immobilization mask to 1 cm for an extremity immobilized in a vacuum-sealed customized cushion.

In general, 100–300 kVp is the typical orthovoltage energy clinically available (Fig. 13.1). Depending on the depth of the target, electron energies available range from 6 to 18 MeV. Unlike orthovoltage, usage of electrons requires bolus

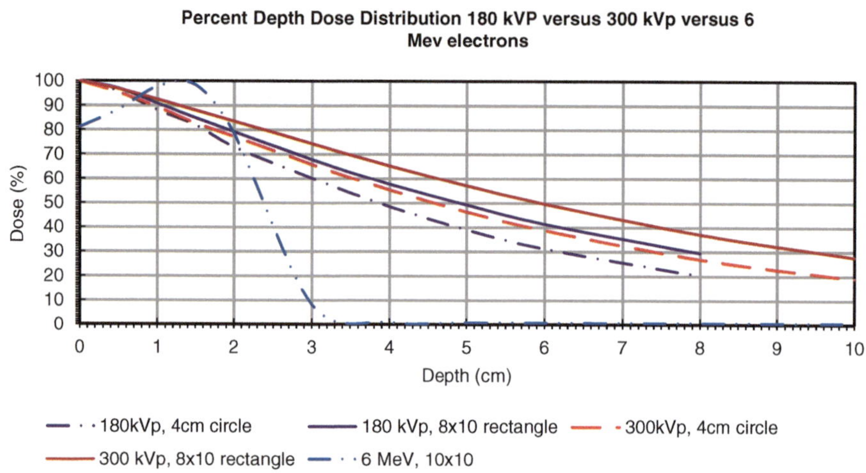

Fig. 13.1 Comparison of 180 vs. 300 kVp. Orthovoltage RT allows near-100% dose at the surface with a rapid drop of dose, thereby minimizing exit dose to deeper organs and structures unaffected by the patient's lymphoma. The dose distribution is dependent on the treatment field size and energy. In comparison, electron dose builds up, reaching a maximum dose 1–2 cm into tissue. To avoid skin sparing, tissue equivalent bolus is required to build up the electron dose to the surface. (Figure courtesy of Cross Cancer Institute Physics Department)

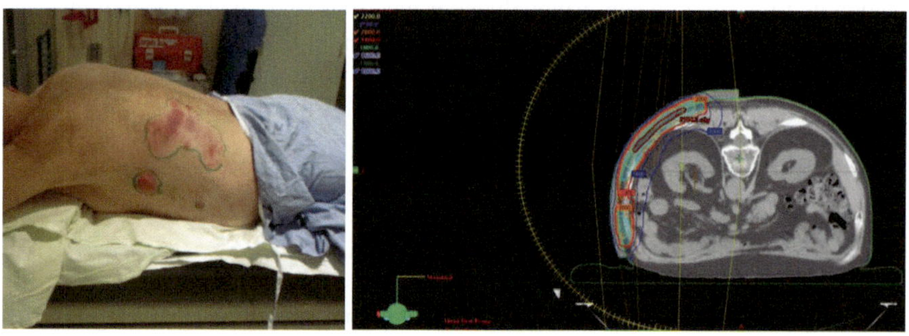

Fig. 13.2 MF lesion left posterior flank treated with VMAT. Recurrence of MF lesions on left posterior flank, a mix of plaques and patches primarily in the larger outlined area. The circular lesion along the posterior axillary line is more in keeping with a tumorous deposit. The inked outline demarcates where wires were placed to help localize the tumor on CT simulation. Patient was treated with VMAT

application to ensure ≥95% dose on skin surface. For single beam (direct orthovoltage or direct electrons), the field encompasses the GTV, CTV, PTV, and penumbra.

At times, more advanced delivery techniques are required for treatment planning. Larger lesions or multiple small lesions spread over a large volume of skin may not be adequately covered by orthovoltage or electrons. Other options such as IMRT/VMAT with bolus or brachytherapy could be considered (Fig. 13.2).

Table 13.2 Typical radiotherapy doses used for cutaneous lymphomas

Primary cutaneous T cell lymphoma	Dose fractionation
Unilesional radical radiotherapy	20–30 Gy in 1.8–2 Gy daily fractions
Total skin electron beam therapy	8–36 Gy in 1.8–2 Gy fractions[a]
Local palliation	4 Gy in 2 daily fractions; 8–12 Gy (e.g., 8 Gy in 1 fraction, 12 Gy in 3 daily fractions)

[a]Details regarding total skin electron beam therapy can be found in the literature as some institutions are treating patients in <1.8 Gy per fraction now [8, 9]. It is beyond the scope of this work

The International Lymphoma Radiation Oncology Group (ILROG) published guidelines for primary cutaneous lymphoma [7]. Table 13.2 summarizes typical dose fractionation schedules for PCTCL.

In general, 20–30 Gy in 2 Gy daily fractions is usually sufficient for achieving in-field tumor control. We routinely prescribe 20 Gy in 10 fractions at our institution. Doses less than 20 Gy may lead to earlier recurrences. While there is no randomized controlled trial assessing the ideal dose of RT in these patients, small studies have shown 10-year local control rates up to 75% with 20 Gy in 2 Gy daily fractions [10]. Further, 20 Gy in 2 Gy daily fractions allows for re-treatment with minimal chronic side effects from RT [7]. However, effective palliation can be achieved in as little as 2–4 Gy × 2 fractions with response rates >90% [11]. As per the ILROG published guidelines, we routinely use at least 2 cm margins to ensure adequate coverage of cutaneous lesions.

Examples of Mycosis Fungoides Treatment

Example 1. Patient developed a lesion along the left posterior flank (Fig. 13.3a). MF was treated with 300 kVp orthovoltage radiotherapy, with a dose of 20 Gy in 10 fractions using a 6x8 cm applicator, with a field source distance (FSD) of 50 cm. While patient achieved a complete response following treatment, he subsequently developed satellite lesions approximately 1 year later and was then treated again with 20 Gy in 10 fractions utilizing 300 kVp orthovoltage via a 12 × 12 cm applicator at an FSD of 30 cm (Fig. 13.3a, b).

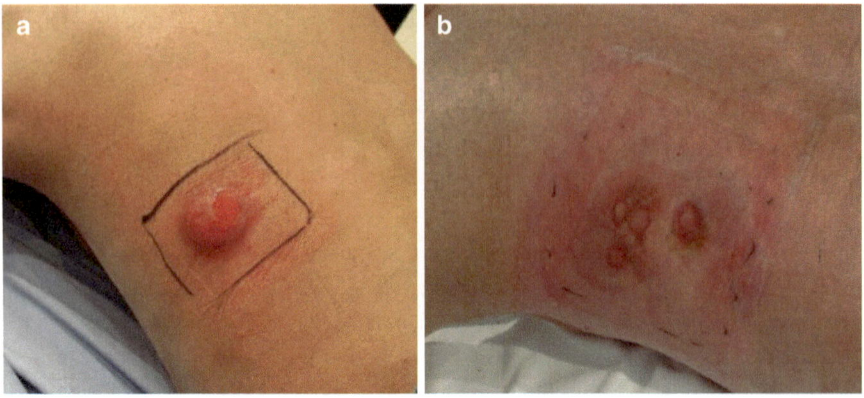

Fig. 13.3 Patient with stage IIB MF treated with orthovoltage. A 65-year-old patient with stage IIB MF was diagnosed nearly 10 years ago via a punch biopsy of a forehead lesion that was positive for CD3 and negative for CD7 and CD56. PET-CT was undertaken at the time to rule out systemic involvement. He had previously been treated with topical steroids, psoralen and ultraviolet light (PUVA), and interferon

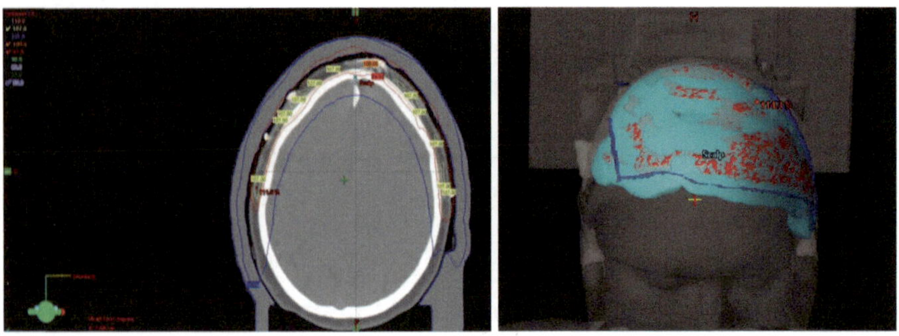

Fig. 13.4 VMAT used to treeat confluent cutaneous lymphoma scalp. Following treatment of the above lesions, patient subsequently developed numerous scalp lesions. The lesions presented at different phases from patches to tumors with varying degrees of depth to the lesions. Therefore, VMAT was used to provide more conformal coverage. He was treated using 6 MV photons with 2 hemi-arcs and daily bolus (Fig. 13.4). The furthermost border of the lesions was outlined using a radio-opaque wire to guide with GTV delineation. A 1.0 cm bolus was used to ensure appropriate surface dose (Fig. 13.4). He was treated with 20 Gy in 10 fractions. The patient is currently in remission

Example 2. The following is a 46-year-old male who developed MF of the sole of right foot (Fig. 13.5a). Localized disease treated with electron beam radiotherapy received a dose of 20 Gy delivered over 2 weeks. Figure 13.5b shows response to treatment 5 months after radiation.

In cases of more widespread cutaneous lesions (T2–T3 disease), total skin electron beam therapy (TSEBT) may provide a more comprehensive tumor coverage. However, the treatment is not offered in every center and can be both resource intensive and time consuming. The original Stanford technique required treatment in various positions per day over a course of approximately 3 months: 36 Gy over 9–12 weeks, 3 fields per day using 9 MeV electrons. A total of 6 positions were

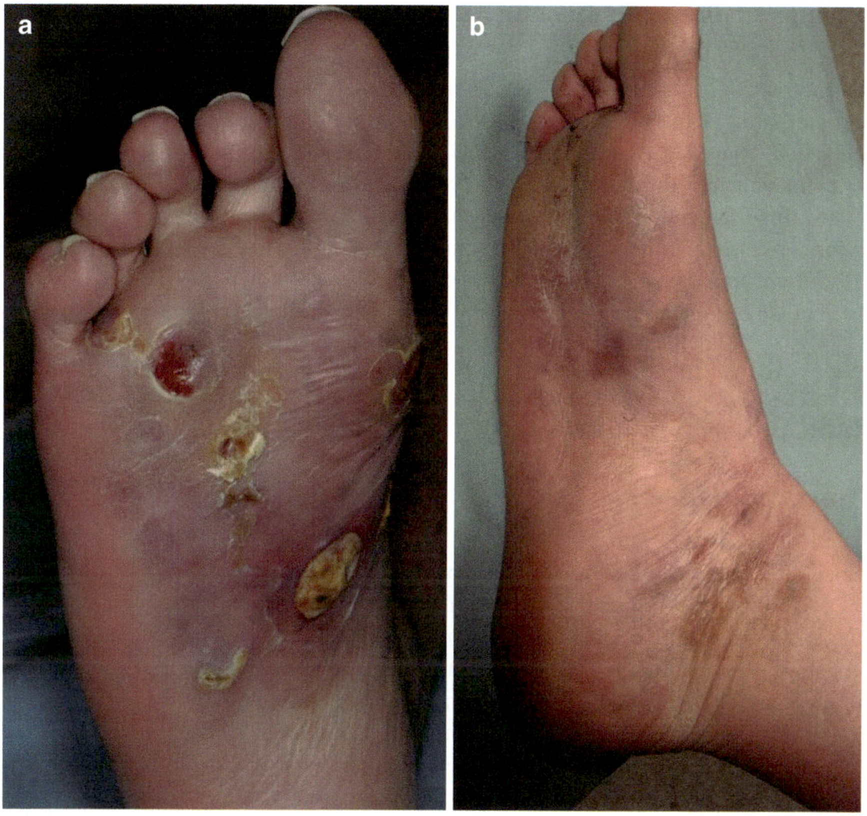

Fig. 13.5 Patient with ulcerated MF sole of Foot. Some patients may present with ulceration of their cutaneous lymphoma rather than tumors or plaques (**a**). Treatment principles are the same and result in excellent healing (**b**)

used, 3 per day. Additional RT was required for the soles of the feet and perineum. Details of this technique can be found in the literature [8, 9]. There were many side effects resulting from treatment including anhidrosis, xerosis, hyperpigmentation, and xerostomia. Modern RT techniques still utilize the same treatment positions, but with a decreased overall dose—10 Gy in 10 fractions, 4 fractions per week, over a course of 2–3 weeks [12]. Areas shielded from TSEBT and thicker lesions were given an additional boost of external beam RT. Overall response rate was 95% with a median duration of response of 6 months. Toxicity profile was much improved compared to the original Stanford technique: 35% alopecia, 15% xerosis, and 10% hyperpigmentation. This modern version of TSEBT allows for reirradiation if patients relapse or progress with fewer side effects.

Once there is concern for systemic involvement of PCTCL, the focus should be on chemotherapy and immunotherapy. A wide variety of agents have been utilized with varying degrees of response rates from interferon and oral retinoids to histone deacetylase inhibitors and monoclonal antibodies. A discussion of these therapies is beyond the scope of this book chapter.

Primary Cutaneous B Cell Lymphomas

In contrast to PCTCL, PCBCL is staged with a TNM system. Like their systemic counterparts, primary cutaneous follicle center lymphoma (PCFCL) and primary cutaneous marginal zone lymphoma (PCMZL) are indolent tumors where the risk of extracutaneous disease is <10% and survival is >95% at 5 years. Primary cutaneous diffuse large B cell lymphoma (PCDLBCL), leg type, is a more aggressive lymphoma that can present with systemic disease in up to 50% of cases [13, 14]. Therefore, appropriate imaging and bone marrow biopsy can be considered if it may help guide treatment in PCDLBCL.

Indications for Radiotherapy

Treatment Planning

Local RT is appropriate for solitary or regional cutaneous T1–T2 lesions. The EORTC/ISCL recommends a minimum of 1–2 cm of healthy skin margin beyond the area of clinically visible erythema or induration is required to ensure adequate coverage. The thickness of the lesions must be defined either clinically or by appropriate imaging to ensure adequate coverage of the depth of the tumor.

Orthovoltage and electrons are the most common modalities used to treat cutaneous lesions. Most lesions can be treated with 6–9 MeV electrons or 100 kV superficial X-rays. Higher energy photons are used for deep and bulky tumors. Bolus is required in electrons or photons and used to prevent skin sparing. VMAT can be an alternative for widespread lesions to achieve better target coverage. In patients with PCDLBCL, leg type, relapse in extra-cutaneous sites is common. Hence, solitary or localized disease is treated initially with R-CHOP (rituximab, cyclophosphamide, adriamycin, vincristine, and prednisone), followed by local RT. If chemotherapy is not tolerated, patient can be treated with RT alone or combined with rituximab [15].

Dose

The NCCN recommends that a dose of 24–40 Gy in 1.8–2 Gy daily fractions is sufficient for tumor control for PCBCL [7, 16–18]. Table 13.3 summarizes typical dose fractionation schedules for PCBCL. Like PCTCL, palliation can be achieved with low-dose (2 Gy × 2) RT with a response rate of 86%, but worse complete response rates (86% vs. 29%, *p* 0.007) [19]. The EORTC and the International Society for Cutaneous Lymphomas (ISCL) recommend a dose range of 20–36 Gy for PCMZL

Table 13.3 Common dose fractionations for primary cutaneous B cell lymphomas

Primary cutaneous B cell lymphoma	Dose fractionation
Primary cutaneous follicle center, marginal zone, anaplastic large cell	Radical: 24–40 Gy in 1.8–2 Gy daily fractions Palliative: 4 Gy in 2 daily fractions
Primary cutaneous diffuse large B cell lymphoma, leg type	Radical: 36–40 Gy in 1.8–2 Gy daily fractions Palliative: 4 Gy in 2 daily fractions

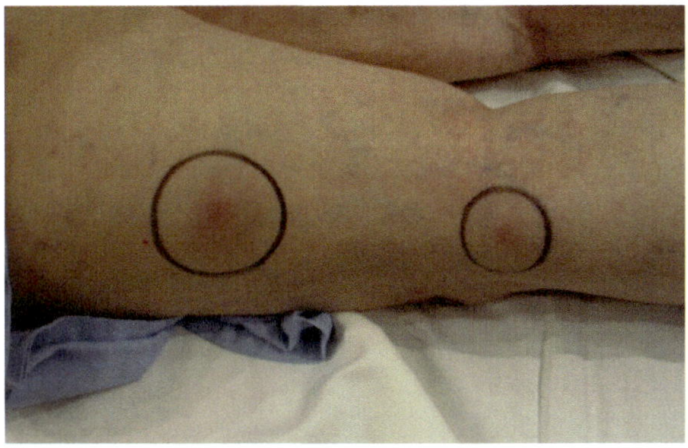

Fig. 13.6 A case of PCMZL treated with orthovoltage

and 30 Gy for PCFCL [7]. A higher dose of local RT is recommended for primary cutaneous diffuse large B cell lymphoma (PCDLBCL) of 40 Gy.

A 77-year-old female with a long-standing history of primary cutaneous marginal zone lymphoma (PCMZL) was treated with multiple courses of RT (electrons and orthovoltage) to lesions on the scalp, forearm, and legs. A positron-emission tomography-computed tomography (PET-CT) scan demonstrated no systemic disease. Her most recent course of RT was to two lesions on the posterior left leg (Fig. 13.6). The larger lesion was treated with a 6.0 cm circular applicator, FSD 30 cm, 200 kVp. The inferior, smaller lesion was treated with a 4.0 cm circular applicator, FSD 30 cm, 200 kVp. Both lesions were treated with 24 Gy in 12 fractions prescribed to Dmax. Unfortunately, she did not develop a complete response to RT and began to develop new cutaneous lesions. With the extent of her disease, she was started on rituximab and bendamustine chemotherapy.

Outcomes

Overall, most patients will achieve a complete remission following RT [11, 17]. However, while primary cutaneous follicle center lymphoma (PCFCL) has an excellent response rate, a small number of patients may develop recurrence. Recurrences in cutaneous indolent B cell lymphomas generally occur on the skin. In contrast, PCDLBCL has the worst prognosis with higher rate of recurrences (skin or extra-cutaneous). Senff et al. reported on 153 PCBCL patients treated with RT; 5-year relapse-free survival in patients presenting with PCDLBCL was only 36% compared to 70% in PCFCL [17, 18]. Therefore, while RT is still the mainstay of treatment in solitary cutaneous PCDLBCL, it is often given in conjunction with rituximab-based systemic therapy. In one study of 136 patients with PCBCL, RT improved time to progression, and while not statistically significant, rituximab improved survival in PCDLBCL cases [20]. Further analyses support the use of rituximab-based chemotherapy to improve survival in PCDLBCL patients [21]. In the same way as generalized PCTCL is treated with systemic agents, for generalized skin disease in PCBCL (or patients presenting with recurrences or systemic disease), chemotherapy is utilized. Like their systemic counterparts, selected patients with indolent PCBCL may be treated with rituximab-based chemotherapy. Innovative chemotherapy and immunotherapy are currently being investigated to treat PCBCL [13].

References

1. Cai ZR, Chen ML, Weinstock MA, Kim YH, Novoa RA, Linos E. Incidence trends of primary cutaneous T-cell lymphoma in the US from 2000 to 2018: a SEER population data analysis. JAMA Oncol. 2022;8(11):1690–2.
2. Willemze R, Hodak E, Zinzani PL, Specht L, Ladetto M. ESMO Guidelines Committee primary cutaneous lymphomas: ESMO Clinical Practice Guidelines for diagnosis, treatment and follow-up. Ann Oncol. 2018;29(Suppl 4):iv30–40.
3. Surmanowicz P, Doherty S, Sivanand A, Parvinnejad N, et al. The clinical spectrum of primary cutaneous CD4+ small/medium sized pleomorphic T cell lymphoproliferative disorder: an updated systemic literature review and case series. Dermatology. 2021;237(4):618–28.
4. Kim YH. Management with topical nitrogen mustard in mycosis fungoides. Dermatol Ther. 2003;16(4):288–98.
5. El-Mofty M, Mostafa WZ, Bosseila M, et al. A large scale analytical study on efficacy of different photo(chemo)therapeutic modalities in the treatment of psoriasis, vitiligo and mycosis fungoides. Dermatol Ther. 2010;23(4):428–34.
6. Heald P, Mehlmauer M, Martin AG, Crowley CA, Yocum RC, Reich SD, Worldwide Bexarotene Study Group. Topical bexarotene therapy for patients with refractory or persistent early-stage cutaneous T-cell lymphoma: results of the phase III clinical trial. J Am Acad Dermatol. 2003;49(5):801–15.
7. Specht L, Dabaja B, Illidge T, Wilson LD, Hoppe RT, International Lymphoma Radiation Oncology Group. Modern radiation therapy for primary cutaneous lymphomas: field and dose guidelines from the International Lymphoma Radiation Oncology Group. Int J Radiat Oncol Biol Phys. 2015;92(1):32–9.
8. Hoppe RT, Fuks Z, Bagshaw MA. The rationale for curative radiotherapy in mycosis fungoides. Int J Radiat Oncol Biol Phys. 1977;2(9–10):843–51.
9. Ysebaert L, Truc G, Dalac S, et al. Ultimate results of radiation therapy for T1–T2 mycosis fungoides (including reirradiation). Int J Radiat Oncol Biol Phys. 2004;58(4):1128–34.

10. Wilson LD, Kacinski BM, Jones GW. Local superficial radiotherapy in the management of minimal stage IA cutaneous T-cell lymphoma (mycosis fungoides). Int J Radiat Oncol Biol Phys. 1998;40(1):109–15.
11. Neelis KJ, Schimmel EC, Vermeer MH, Senff NJ, Willemze R, Noordijk EM. Low-dose palliative radiotherapy for cutaneous B- and T-cell lymphomas. Int J Radiat Oncol Biol Phys. 2009;74(1):154–8.
12. Kamstrup MR, Gniadecki R, Iversen L, Skov L, Petersen PM, Loft A, Specht L. Low-dose (10-Gy) total skin electron beam therapy for cutaneous T-cell lymphoma: an open clinical study and pooled data analysis. Int J Radiat Oncol Biol Phys. 2015;92(1):138–43.
13. Krenitsky A, Klager S, Hatch L, Sarriera-Lazaro C, Chen PL, Seminario-Vidal L. Update in diagnosis and management of primary cutaneous B-cell lymphomas. Am J Clin Dermatol. 2022;23(5):689–706.
14. Hristov AC, Tejasvi T, Wilcox RA. Cutaneous B-cell lymphomas: 2021 update on diagnosis, risk-stratification, and management. Am J Hematol. 2020;96(10):1313–28.
15. Heinzerling LM, Urbanek M, Funk JO, et al. Reduction of tumor burden and stabilization of disease by systemic therapy with anti-CD20 antibody (rituximab) in patients with primary cutaneous B-cell lymphoma. Cancer. 2000;89:1835–44.
16. NCCN Clinical Practice Guidelines in Oncology, Non-Hodgkin's Lymphomas Version 1.2015. http://www.nccn.org/professionals/physician_gls/pdf/nhl.pdf.
17. Senff NJ, Hoefnagel JJ, Neelis KJ, Vermeer MH, Noordijk EM, Willemze R, Dutch Cutaneous Lymphoma Group. Results of radiotherapy in 153 primary cutaneous B-cell lymphomas classified according to the WHO–EORTC classification. Arch Dermatol. 2007;143(12):1520–6.
18. Senff NJ, Noordijk EM, Kim YH, et al. European Organization for Research and Treatment of Cancer and International Society for Cutaneous Lymphoma consensus recommendations for the management of cutaneous B-cell lymphomas. Blood. 2008;112(5):1600–9.
19. Oertel M, Elsayad K, Weishaupt C, Steinbrink K, Eich HT. De-escalated radiotherapy for indolent primary cutaneous B-cell lymphoma. Strahlenther Onkol. 2020;196(2):126–31.
20. Hamilton SN, Wai ES, Tan K, Alexander C, Gascoyne RD, Connors JM. Treatment and outcomes in patients with primary cutaneous B-cell lymphoma: the BC Cancer Agency experience. Int J Radiat Oncol Biol Phys. 2013;87(4):719–25.
21. Grange F, Maubec E, Bagot M, Beylot-Barry M, et al. Treatment of cutaneous B-cell lymphoma, leg type, with age-adapted combinations of chemotherapies and rituximab. Arch Dermatol. 2009;145(3):329–30.

Chapter 14
Regional Radiotherapy in Head and Neck Non-melanoma Skin Cancer

Justin Smith and Sandro V. Porceddu

The majority (>90%) of non-melanoma skin cancers (NMSCs) are adequately treated with either surgery or radiotherapy (RT). A subgroup of patients will present with locoregionally advanced NMSC, which includes higher grade primary tumours (T3–4) and/or those with metastatic regional disease. Regional metastasis occurs in approximately 5% of patients with cSCC. The majority (80–90%) of cSCCs occur in the head and neck region and the intraparotid nodes followed by cervical nodes are the most frequently involved [1]. Spread of basal cell carcinoma (BCC) to nodes is rare, with an estimated incidence of <1%. The presence of regional nodal metastases confers a lower overall survival and disease-specific survival, with survival rate reported in the literature between 50 and 70% [2]. Given that NMSC most commonly occurs in the head and neck region, this site will be the primary focus of this chapter. For the purposes of this chapter, NMSC will be referred to as cSCC and BCC.

The current standard of care for patients with metastatic nodal NMSC involves surgical dissection followed by adjuvant regional RT. RT alone is generally recommended in patients who are deemed inoperable, those who refuse surgery or patients

J. Smith
Radiation Oncology Department, Princess Alexandra Hospital, Brisbane, QLD, Australia

Faculty of Medicine, University of QLD, Brisbane, QLD, Australia

College of Medicine and Dentistry, James Cook University, Townsville, QLD, Australia
e-mail: justin.smith3@health.qld.gov.au

S. V. Porceddu (✉)
Faculty of Medicine, University of QLD, Brisbane, QLD, Australia

Peter MacCallum Cancer Centre, Melbourne, VIC, Australia

Department of Radiology, Faculty of Medicine, University of Melbourne,
Melbourne, VIC, Australia
e-mail: sandro.porceddu@petermac.org

K. J. Joseph et al. (eds.), *Radiotherapy in Skin Cancer*,
https://doi.org/10.1007/978-3-031-44316-9_14

requiring palliative treatment. Patients with a clinically node-negative region occasionally may also be considered for elective regional RT depending on the presence or absence of defined high-risk factors. Figure 14.1 shows an algorithm for the management of NMSC patients with nodal involvement in the head and neck region.

A CT scan can be used for staging if regional disease is suspected or thought to be of high risk. Although limited evidence exists, a PET/CT scan is thought to have a higher sensitivity and specificity than CT scan. Figure 14.2 demonstrates the CT and PET/CT appearance of cSCC with regional metastasis to the parotid.

The role of sentinel lymph node biopsy (SLNB) in cSCC has been explored in previous studies and may be helpful in guiding further management options and avoiding neck dissections. However, more evidence is required before incorporation of SLNB into routine clinical practice [1].

Indications for RT

Adjuvant Nodal RT

There is limited high-quality evidence to guide the use of adjuvant post-operative RT (PORT) for regional metastases. Current evidence is based predominantly on retrospective observational cohort studies. Non-immunosuppressed patients with a solitary lymph node <3 cm, without extranodal extension and with adequate excision margins, may be considered for observation rather than adjuvant PORT. A study by Ebrahimi et al. demonstrated good outcomes with surgery alone for these low-risk patients with a single node <3 cm [3]. However, these relatively favourable patients comprise only 5–10% of all patients with metastatic regional cSCC.

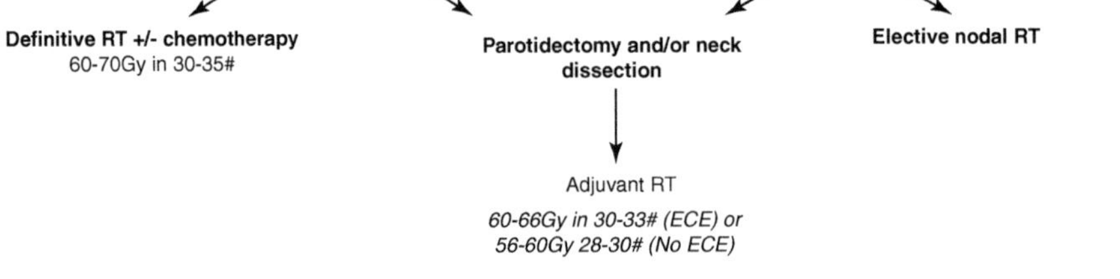

Fig. 14.1 A flow chart for the management of NMSC patients with nodal involvement in the head and neck region

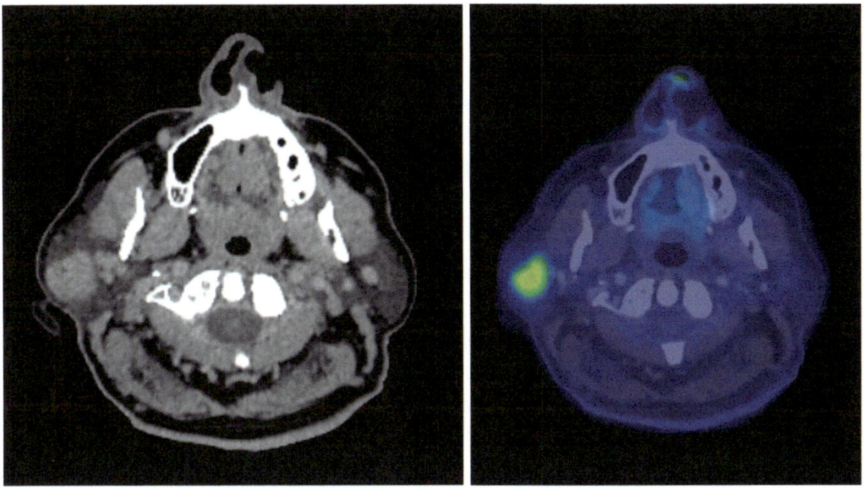

Fig. 14.2 Cutaneous SCC with regional metastasis to the parotid demonstrated on non-contrast CT (left) and PET/CT scan (right)

PORT should be considered in the presence of any of the following

- Single node ≥3 cm
- ≥2 nodes
- Extracapsular extension
- Positive or close (<5 mm) margins
- Perineural invasion
- Dermal or in-transit metastases
- Immunosuppression
- Invasion into surrounding structures (e.g. bone or cranial nerves)

The addition of chemotherapy to PORT has been demonstrated in a randomised control trial to provide no benefit in freedom from regional relapse and disease-free or overall survival [4]. Adjuvant immunotherapy after surgery and RT remains under investigation with a number of randomised control trials ongoing (NCT03969004, NCT03833167).

Definitive RT

Patients unable to undergo surgery can be considered for RT alone, although current non-randomised evidence suggests inferior outcomes with RT alone compared to surgery and PORT [5, 6]. Patients with unresectable regionally advanced disease are often treated with a combination of RT and chemotherapy, although the evidence to support this is limited [7]. The use of immunotherapy in these patients remains an area of active investigation. Interest has also emerged in the role of neoadjuvant immunotherapy for locoregionally advanced but resectable cSCC, with a phase 2 non-randomised study documenting a pathological complete response rate of 51% [8].

Elective Nodal Radiotherapy

Elective treatment may be considered in select cases when the risk of harbouring occult nodal metastases is >15–20%. High-risk features for regional metastases from a primary cSCC include tumour size >2 cm, depth of tumour invasion ≥6 mm, poor differentiation, perineural and lymphovascular invasion and presence of immunosuppression or recurrent disease. Elective nodal treatment may consist of elective nodal dissection or elective regional RT (often treated at the same time when adjuvant RT is required for the primary site). The presence of intraparotid metastases has been shown to confer a risk of occult cervical node involvement with a risk of 20–30%, and cervical nodal irradiation should be considered in these patients that do not undergo an elective upper neck dissection.

Treatment Strategy/Approach

There are no studies directly comparing the benefits of newer highly conformal RT techniques such as IMRT/VMAT in metastatic cutaneous NMSC. However, based on the studies from mucosal head and neck cancer, modern RT techniques such as IMRT/VMAT are recommended for treatment to minimise treatment-related toxicities (Fig. 14.3). Non-IMRT techniques such as 3-dimensional conformal RT can be used provided that appropriate tumour coverage and organ-at-risk (OAR) constraints can be achieved.

Treatment Planning

The Head and Neck Cancer International Group (HNCIG) has developed consensus guidelines outlining the optimal delivery of PORT for cSCC of the head and neck [9]. The high-risk tumour volume (HRTV) is the preoperative gross tumour volume (GTV) transposed onto the planning CT, which is modified to account for post-surgical anatomical changes. The HRTVn is defined as the volume representing the preoperative nodal sites. A boost (HRTVn_Boost) can be considered where there is thought to be a higher microscopic disease burden (such as extranodal extension or positive margins). The high-risk CTV (CTVn_HR) is defined as a minimum 5 mm expansion of the HRTV and may include the entire involved neck nodal levels/basin or the neck dissection/parotidectomy bed. The lesser risk CTV (CTV_LR) is the

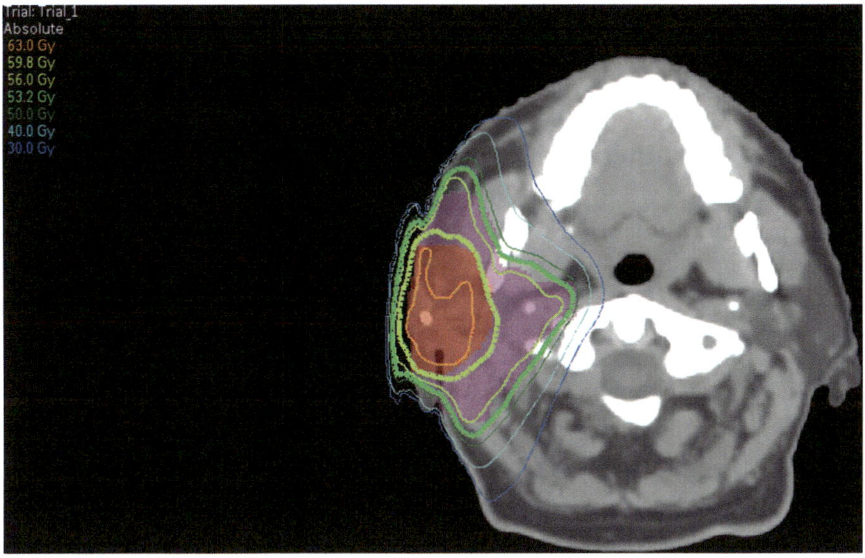

Fig. 14.3 VMAT plan for patient with cSCC and regional metastasis to the parotid gland who underwent surgery and PORT

volume at risk of microscopic disease. A minimum of 5 mm expansion on the CTV is then recommended for the PTV.

Generally, the neck dissection scar does not require full dose to the skin surface (i.e. use of bolus), except when there is gross extranodal extension that extends to the skin or subcutaneous tissues. In this setting, this region needs to be included in the CTV and bolus material used to ensure appropriate coverage.

When RT is used as definitive curative management, the gross disease should be contoured with a minimum 5 mm margin expansion for the CTV and a further 3–5 mm expansion for the PTV.

Dose

For resected nodal disease, the NCCN guidelines recommend a dose of 60–66 Gy in 30–33 fractions when extracapsular extension is present and 56–60 Gy in 28–30 fractions in the absence of extracapsular extension.

Dose to the lower risk neck is 56 Gy in 30 fractions for centres using IMRT/VMAT. For non-IMRT techniques, the recommended dose is 50 Gy in 25 fractions for the surgically unperturbed neck and 54 Gy in 27 fractions for the surgically perturbed neck.

Patients receiving definitive RT for regional involvement are recommended to receive 60–70 Gy in 30–35 fractions, if of good performance status. Shorter hypofractionation schedules such as 30–36 Gy in 5–6 fractions may also be considered in poor performance palliative intent patients.

Regional Radiotherapy in Non-head and Neck Region

Nodal metastases from NMSC, predominantly from cSCC, can also arise in the axilla or groin, although this occurs less commonly than in the head and neck region [10]. Given that this is a relatively uncommon presentation, there is a lack of evidence to guide treatment options in this setting. Management generally follows the principles of nodal metastases of the head and neck region, and treatment usually involves surgical dissection followed by adjuvant RT in patients who are suitable for surgery. There is limited research to guide the recommendations for adjuvant RT after regional lymphadenectomy in the axilla or groin, although it is often recommended in the presence of adverse factors such as multiple positive nodes, close margins or extracapsular extension. Outcomes for patients with nodal metastasis of the axilla or groin are poorer than those with regional disease of the head and neck region, although this is largely based on single-institution retrospective studies. Survival has been variably reported in the literature, but retrospective series have demonstrated 5-year overall survival rates of 33% and 55%, respectively, with a high risk of regional and distant relapse [11, 12].

Treatment-Related Toxicity and Management

The common acute and late side effects of head and neck regional RT vary depending on the site and volume being irradiated. Acute side effects are managed with supportive care during treatment and can include the following:

- Radiation dermatitis
- Fatigue
- Mucositis
- Xerostomia
- Dysgeusia

Late side effects can develop months to years after RT and include

- Lymphoedema
- Hypothyroidism
- Brachial plexopathy
- Xerostomia
- Osteoradionecrosis
- Hearing loss
- Alopecia
- Subcutaneous atrophy and fibrosis

Outcomes

The combination of surgery and PORT has been found to achieve optimal outcomes in patients with regional metastases from NMSC. A retrospective study demonstrated superior outcomes for patients receiving surgery + RT compared to surgery alone for locoregional control (20% vs. 43%) and disease-specific survival (73% vs. 54%) [12]. Five-year disease-specific survival rates vary between studies but are often reported in the literature as between 50 and 70%. The randomised POST (Postoperative Skin Trial) study evaluated outcomes in high-risk locally advanced cSCC, where approximately 50% of patients had extracapsular extension present. This study demonstrated that patients receiving adjuvant RT alone had a similar 5-year locoregional control rate to those receiving adjuvant chemoRT (83% vs. 87%, $P = 0.58$). Five-year overall survival was also similar between the RT-alone and chemoRT groups (76% vs. 79%, $P = 0.86$) [4].

References

1. Porceddu SV, Veness MJ, Guminski A. Nonmelanoma cutaneous head and neck cancer and Merkel cell carcinoma: current concepts, advances, and controversies. J Clin Oncol. 2015;33(29):3338–45. https://doi.org/10.1200/JCO.2014.60.7333.
2. Sahovaler A, Krishnan RJ, Yeh DH, et al. Outcomes of cutaneous squamous cell carcinoma in the head and neck region with regional lymph node metastasis: a systematic review and meta-analysis. JAMA Otolaryngol Head Neck Surg. 2019;145(4):352–60. https://doi.org/10.1001/jamaoto.2018.4515.
3. Ebrahimi A, Clark JR, Lorincz BB, Milross CG, Veness MJ. Metastatic head and neck cutaneous squamous cell carcinoma: defining a low-risk patient. Head Neck. 2012;34(3):365–70. https://doi.org/10.1002/hed.21743.
4. Porceddu SV, Bressel M, Poulsen MG, et al. Postoperative concurrent chemoradiotherapy versus postoperative radiotherapy in high-risk cutaneous squamous cell carcinoma of the head and neck: the randomized phase III TROG 05.01 trial. J Clin Oncol. 2018;36(13):1275–83. https://doi.org/10.1200/jco.2017.77.0941.
5. Hinerman RW, Indelicato DJ, Amdur RJ, et al. Cutaneous squamous cell carcinoma metastatic to parotid-area lymph nodes. Laryngoscope. 2008;118(11):1989–96. https://doi.org/10.1097/MLG.0b013e318180642b.
6. Audet N, Palme CE, Gullane PJ, et al. Cutaneous metastatic squamous cell carcinoma to the parotid gland: analysis and outcome. Head Neck. 2004;26(8):727–32. https://doi.org/10.1002/hed.20048.
7. Likhacheva A, Awan M, Barker CA, et al. Definitive and postoperative radiation therapy for basal and squamous cell cancers of the skin: executive summary of an American Society for Radiation Oncology clinical practice guideline. Pract Radiat Oncol. 2020;10(1):8–20. https://doi.org/10.1016/j.prro.2019.10.014.
8. Gross ND, Miller DM, Khushalani NI, et al. Neoadjuvant cemiplimab for stage II to IV cutaneous squamous-cell carcinoma. N Engl J Med. 2022;387(17):1557–68. https://doi.org/10.1056/NEJMoa2209813.
9. Porceddu SV, Daniels C, Yom SS, et al. Head and neck cancer international group (HNCIG) consensus guidelines for the delivery of postoperative radiation therapy in complex cutane-

ous squamous cell carcinoma of the head and neck (cSCCHN). Int J Radiat Oncol Biol Phys. 2020;107(4):641–51. https://doi.org/10.1016/j.ijrobp.2020.03.024.
10. Bucknell NW, Gyorki DE, Bressel M, et al. Cutaneous squamous cell carcinoma metastatic to the axilla and groin: outcomes and prognostic factors. Australas J Dermatol. 2022;63(1):43–52. https://doi.org/10.1111/ajd.13739.
11. Pang G, Look Hong NJ, Paull G, et al. Squamous cell carcinoma with regional metastasis to axilla or groin lymph nodes: a multicenter outcome analysis. Ann Surg Oncol. 2019;26(13):4642–50. https://doi.org/10.1245/s10434-019-07743-8.
12. Veness MJ, Morgan GJ, Palme CE, Gebski V. Surgery and adjuvant radiotherapy in patients with cutaneous head and neck squamous cell carcinoma metastatic to lymph nodes: combined treatment should be considered best practice. Laryngoscope. 2005;115(5):870–5. https://doi.org/10.1097/01.MLG.0000158349.64337.ED.

Part III
Brachytherapy for Skin Cancer

Chapter 15
Skin Brachytherapy: Overview

Michael E. Kasper and Hina Saeed

Introduction

Cutaneous squamous cell carcinoma (cSCC) and basal cell carcinoma (BCC) are the most common types of keratinocyte carcinoma (KC), formerly known as non-melanoma skin cancer (NMSC). Although surgery is considered as the definitive treatment, radiotherapy (RT) using high-dose-rate (HDR) brachytherapy (BT) has been used more and more over the past decade for the treatment of early-stage KC. This chapter is an overview of the various skin BT techniques including HDR-BT using standard surface applicators and custom surface molds, electronic BT (eBT), and interstitial BT.

The history of external beam RT and BT in treating KC dates back to the beginning of the twentieth century, shortly after Roentgen discovered X-rays in 1895. James Sequeira described successful treatment of 12 "skin cancers" in 1901, and in 1902, Marie Curie provided radium for the first BT application to treat skin cancers. Grenz rays were developed in the 1920s, followed by superficial and orthovoltage-generating treatment machines. Radioactive surface molds and interstitial BT, along with superficial and orthovoltage RT, were the established radiation modalities for many years in treating KC. With the advent of the linear accelerator in the 1950s and increasing availability of electron beam therapy, treatment with surface and

M. E. Kasper (✉)
Department of Radiation Oncology, Lynn Cancer Institute, Boca Raton Regional Hospital, Boca Raton, FL, USA

Baptist Health South Florida, South Florida, USA
e-mail: mkasper@baptisthealth.net

H. Saeed
Department of Radiation Oncology, Lynn Cancer Institute, Boca Raton Regional Hospital, Baptist Health South Florida, Boca Raton, FL, USA
e-mail: hina.saeed@baptisthealth.net

K. J. Joseph et al. (eds.), *Radiotherapy in Skin Cancer*,
https://doi.org/10.1007/978-3-031-44316-9_15

interstitial BT declined. However, the development in the late 1960s of the HDR-BT afterloader greatly improved radiation protection and simplified treatment delivery. HDR-BT is now widely accepted, and there is an increasing body of literature supporting the advantages of hypofractionation and HDR [1].

The advantages for skin BT as a treatment option for KC are due to its ability to deposit a significantly higher dose within the tumor with adequate sparing of adjacent normal structures, compared to external beam radiotherapy (EBRT). Surface BT is a safe, effective, less invasive, and well-tolerated treatment modality, especially among elderly patients who may not tolerate radical surgery or lengthy treatment with EBRT. The treatment is very convenient since it involves fewer treatment fractions and results in excellent local control in the range of 90–98% with desirable cosmetic and functional outcomes [2, 3].

Indications for BT

Surgical options are most often utilized in the treatment of KC, but primary and adjuvant RT can make a major difference in outcomes. In many cases, RT can increase cure rates, and in others improve functional and cosmetic results.

BT is used as a primary modality, adjuvant therapy after surgery, or treatment of recurrent lesions after EBRT. Surface BT is more commonly used for small lesions with a maximum diameter of 20 mm and the maximum depth of invasion of 3–4 mm located at, or just below, the skin surface (measured by punch biopsy and/or ultrasonography). Lesions deeper than 5 mm are best treated by interstitial BT [3, 4].

Tumors with high-risk pathologic features (morpheaform, sclerosing, mixed, infiltrative, or micronodular growth pattern or perineural invasion) or that are poorly defined should not be treated with BT.

Bone invasion is an absolute contraindication for BT. Other contraindications are genetic diseases such as ataxia telangiectasia, xeroderma pigmentosa, or other related diseases of DNA repair; suspected extension into the orbit or deep extension along fascial planes; and perineural invasion [3]. Relative contraindications are collagen vascular diseases, basal cell nevus syndrome, and other diseases where ionizing radiation is inappropriate. BT is usually limited to older patients (>50 years) decreasing the possibility of long-term sequela or secondary malignancies.

Treatment Strategy/Approach

BT delivers radiation close to or within the tumor or surgical scar, exposing very little normal tissue. Margins are smaller with BT resulting in a more precise treatment. This improved targeting allows higher, more effective radiation doses to be delivered over shorter treatment times. For instance, a typical course of RT that takes 4–8 weeks of daily treatment can be completed with BT in as little as 1–3 weeks [5, 6]. As in superficial and orthovoltage RT, there is no "buildup region" with skin surface BT, so bolus is not necessary. Although many of the advantages of

BT can be duplicated with superficial therapy or orthovoltage RT, BT provides several benefits over traditional RT as mentioned before.

BT is described by the position of the isotope in relationship to the tumor, the isotope used, and the dose rate. For KC, the most common types of BT are small surface applicators, surface molds and flaps, and interstitial BT. Electronic BT delivery systems have recently become commercially available as well. The small applicators and surface molds and flaps most often utilize Ir-192 HDR remote afterloaders, although Co-60 and, less frequently, Yb-169 are also used. Interstitial BT employs a wide range of isotopes and dose rates. Ir-192 is most commonly used, although I-125, Pd-103, and Cs-131 are utilized as well. Dose rates can be either low dose rate (LDR) (0.4–2 Gray (Gy)/h), HDR (>12 Gy/h), or pulsed dose rate (PDR; up to 1 Gy/pulse).

The small, cup-shaped, surface applicators such as the Leipzig and Valencia applicators (Elekta and Varian) are shielded applicators of high atom number (high-Z material) placed directly on the skin and attached to an afterloader. These applicators, with a single dwell position, have diameters of 10–50 mm and source-to-surface distance (SSD) of 5–15 mm. Treatment time is approximately 2–15 min depending on the size of the applicator, presence of a flattening filter, and source strength. Proper placement with complete contact on a flat surface is critical to avoid an air gap, which can result in significant underdosage. Too much pressure can result in hypoxic change to the target tissue or overdosage by compressing tissue. The La Fe-ITIC™ template simplifies targeting for the small applicators and helps to avoid inter-fraction setup errors. The La Fe-ITIC template (Fig. 15.1) is a see-through plastic tool to allow measuring and outlining margins on the skin [2].

Electronic BT (eBT) treatment of KC is based on the technical and clinical data obtained from radionuclide skin surface BT and the small skin surface applicators developed over the past 30 years. Radiation is generated by an electronic source with energies ranging from 50 to 69.5 kV, requiring minimal shielding. Applicator diameters range from 10 to 50 mm. The SSD for the three commercially available

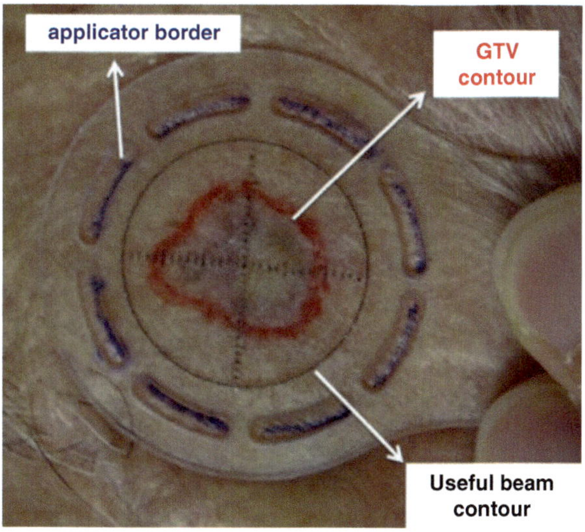

Fig. 15.1 La Fe-ITIC template (courtesy of Jose Perez-Calatayud, with permission)

systems, Xoft Axxent, Zeiss INTRABEAM, and Elekta Esteya, ranges from 16.9 to 60 mm. Treatment times are similar to the radionuclide-based small applicators, and proper placement with complete contact on a flat surface is essential [4].

Surface molds and flaps can be custom made or prefabricated. They are designed to deliver a homogeneous dose to the skin surface by closely following the contour of the skin and securing the catheters at a fixed distance. Molds have traditionally been constructed of soft materials such as wax with carefully placed parallel and equidistant catheters (Fig. 15.2). 3D printing of thermoplastic molds conforming to CT scans of the skin surface has significantly improved and simplified the construction of custom molds, essentially eliminating the variation previously seen with manual construction.

Flaps are commercially available flexible mesh-style molds housing catheters at a set geometry. Catheters are usually elevated 3–5 mm from the skin surface by the mold or flap and separated by 10 mm. CT planning is performed using catheter reconstruction and computerized algorithms, allowing dose optimization to a depth of approximately 5 mm. Although molds and flaps can be used for small or large lesions, flaps are produced as large sheets (up to 24 cm) and are usually used for larger, superficial lesions. The flaps are reusable and can be cut to size.

Interstitial BT has the longest track record of all the BT techniques for treatment of KC but it is the least utilized. Interstitial BT is indicated in lesions of ≥5 mm thickness and in some challenging anatomic locations where surface applicators would not be physically possible. By definition, the procedure is invasive and requires local or general anesthesia. As in all interstitial BT, there is a steep learning curve in mastering the procedure. A catheter array is placed encompassing the lesion and a margin in single or multiple planes. Catheters should ideally be placed 3–5 mm below the skin surface to avoid skin necrosis, ulceration, or late skin changes such as telangiectasias. Catheters in the same plane should be separated by 8–12 mm, and if multiple planes are required, as may be needed for thicker lesions, 5–7 mm separation is optimal [3, 6].

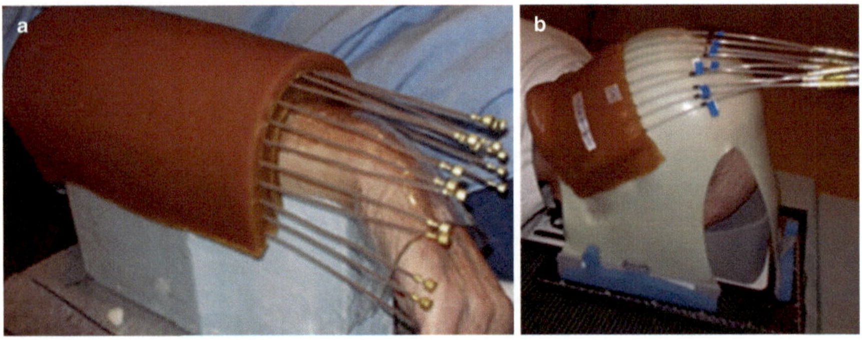

Fig. 15.2 Custom wax molds for (**a**) forearm and (**b**) scalp. The wax material can be shaped to the contour of the external anatomy (**a**) or mounted on an immobilizing mask (**b**). Catheters are placed at uniform separation of about 10 mm along the plane of treatment

Treatment Margins

Treatment margins in BT should be considered in the context of the minimally recommended surgical margins. Broadland and Zitelli recommended a minimum of 4 mm margins for Mohs resection of low-risk lesions and 6 mm for high-risk lesions to expect a 95% or greater likelihood of complete extirpation (e.g., gross tumor volume (GTV) → clinical target volume (CTV)) [7]. Surface BT requires an additional margin for setup uncertainty. For small applicators and eBT, this is usually as little as 2 mm in addition to the original 4–6 mm (CTV → planning target volume (PTV)). When treating poorly demarcated lesions and variants known to require wider margins, an additional 5 mm at a minimum is recommended.

Flaps and molds are usually utilized for somewhat larger lesions, and an additional 5 mm in addition to the original 4–6 mm margin is recommended. For poorly demarcated, poorly differentiated, or variants known to require wider margins, up to an additional 10 mm margin should be considered. Dermoscopy and high-frequency skin ultrasound are sometimes used to help delineate margins [6, 7]. Interstitial BT is planned to fully encompass the lesion with margins of at least 5–10 mm. Catheters are placed along or beyond edges of visible tumor to ensure coverage. The CTV generally equals PTV for interstitial BT [3, 5, 6].

Clinical judgment is required in critical anatomic locations where it is difficult or not possible to achieve the recommended margins. Treating with smaller margins is a compromise that must be weighed against the disadvantages of alternatives, if any.

A minimum of 1 mm additional margin should be considered for microscopic extension at depth. Wider margins are used for lesions with high-risk features such as close or positive margins. Tumor depth is often judged clinically. The dose from small applicators is usually specified to a maximum of 3 mm to limit surface dose, with 4 mm receiving approximately 90% of the specified dose. Exophytic lesions are often shaved at biopsy, limiting lesion thickness and rendering the lesion amenable to treatment with a 1 mm margin at depth. Endophytic lesions are more difficult to assess and should be further evaluated. High-frequency skin ultrasound (HFUS), with ultrasound frequencies of 18–100 MHz, is a useful imaging tool for lesions thought to extend deeper than 2–3 mm (Fig. 15.3). [2] Multiple studies have shown excellent correlation of tumor depth between HFUS and pathologic specimens. Video-dermoscopy in combination with HFUS can increase the accuracy of margin delineation and estimation of depth of invasion [6, 8].

The treatment depth of surface molds and flaps is specified based on CT imaging. If the lesion is thought to possibly extend deeply, consideration of additional imaging with HFUS and/or MRI should be entertained.

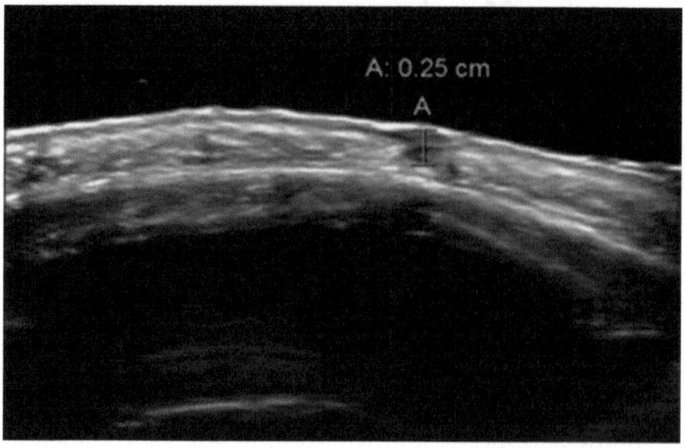

Fig. 15.3 2.5 mm nodular lesion imaged with 18 MHz high-resolution ultrasound unit (Courtesy of Z Ouhib et al. with permission)

Treatment Planning and Dose

Traditional external beam RT dose schedules for KC have been 50–66 Gy over 4–7 weeks at standard daily doses per fraction of 2–2.5 Gy. Hypofractionated courses were occasionally given for smaller lesions and palliative cases. Early interstitial and surface BT treatments often utilized hypofractionated schedules. More recently, with standardized surface molds and small surface applicators, hypofractionated schedules have become standard.

A 2016 survey demonstrated a wide range of preferred schedules among surveyed respondents [9]. Likhacheva et al. studied contemporary practice patterns of care among radiation oncologists who use skin surface BT for the treatment of KC. There was no consensus regarding treatment planning, dosimetric constraints, or specified dose. Ouhib et al. in 2015 provided a literature overview and best practices for skin BT, including a standard reference for treatment planning and patient evaluation tools [3]. Guidelines for clinical and dosimetric planning, appropriate margin delineation, and applicator selection were proposed. Dose prescription, dose fractionation schedules, and prescription depth were also addressed. Subsequent recommendations from the American Brachytherapy Society (ABS) and GEC-ESTRO were also published. All have been consistent in recommending a minimum radiobiological dose of 60 Gy10 EQD2 for BCC and 65 Gy10 EQD2 for cSCC [3, 5, 6].

For surface applicators such as the Leipzig, Valencia, and eBT applicators (Figs. 15.4 and 15.5), frequently used dose schedules include 40 Gy/8 fractions and 42 Gy/6 fractions delivered every other day or twice weekly. By convention, doses are typically specified at 3 mm. Surface doses therefore range from 125 to 150% of the prescribed dose. Approximately 90% of the prescribed dose will extend to 4 mm depth, with rapid falloff at additional depth.

For flaps and custom molds (Figs. 15.6, 15.7, 15.8, 15.9), common doses are 40 Gy/10 fractions and 40 Gy/8 fractions, delivered every other day or twice weekly. Higher fractionation schedules are sometimes used when treating larger volumes

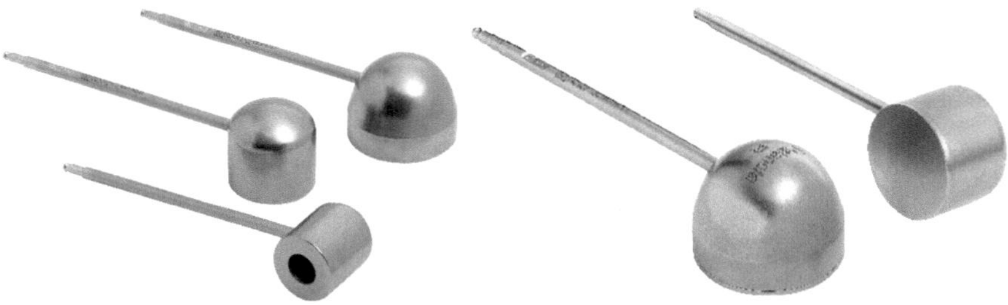

Fig. 15.4 Elekta's Leipzig (left) and Valencia (right) applicators (Images courtesy of Elekta)

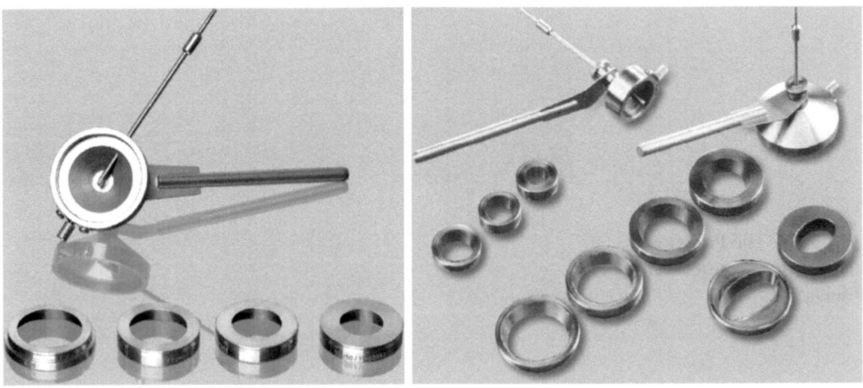

Fig. 15.5 Varian's surface applicator set (Leipzig-style cone is shown on the left). (Images courtesy of Varian)

Fig. 15.6 The Varian catheter flap (Images courtesy of Varian)

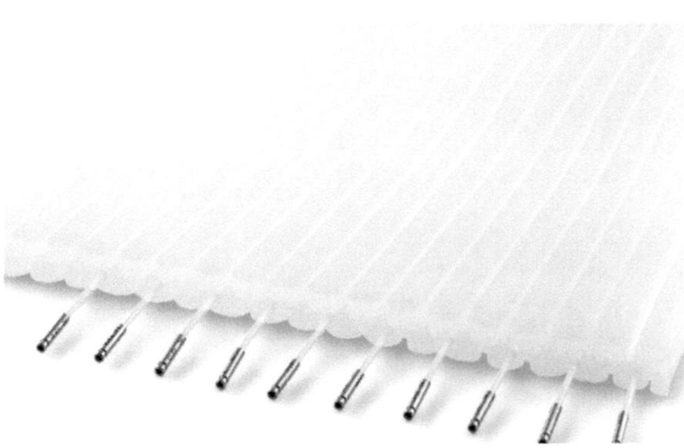

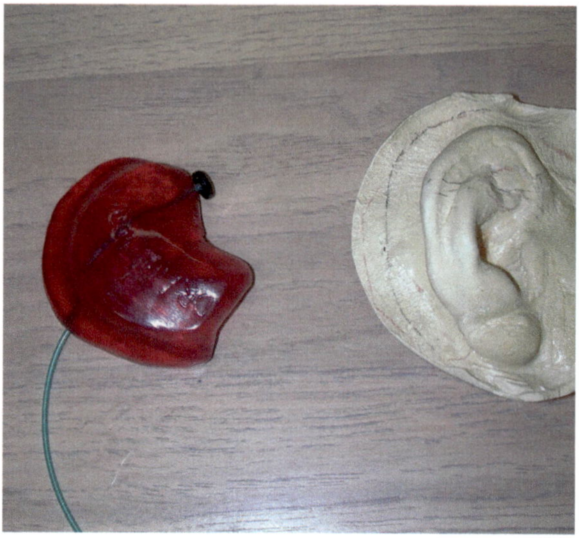

Fig. 15.7 In-house custom mold

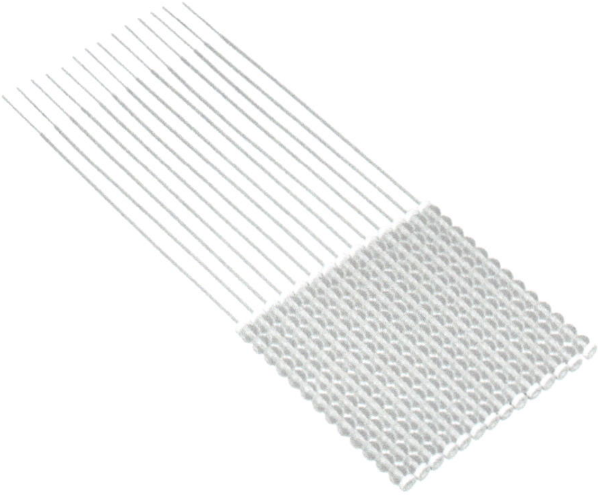

Fig. 15.8 The Freiburg flap (Images courtesy of Elekta)

and more sensitive areas such as the pretibial skin. Doses are typically specified up to a maximum depth of 5 mm based on CT treatment planning.

Due to larger volumes usually included in flap and mold treatments, surface doses are often limited to 125% (Fig. 15.9).

Reported interstitial dose schedules are more variable, often based on dosimetric specifications. Specified doses range from 30 to 55 Gy in 8–10 fractions BID.

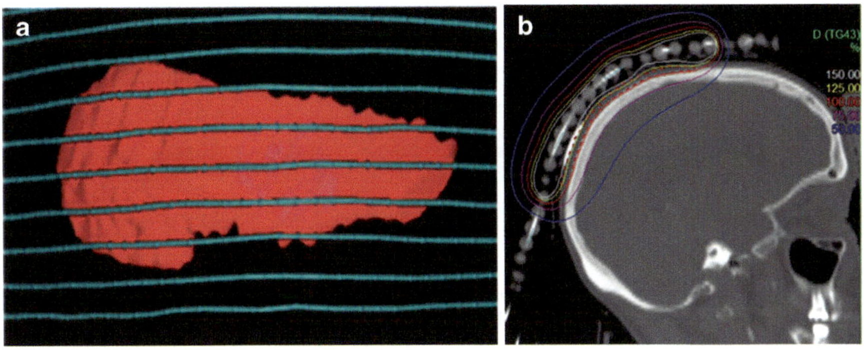

Fig. 15.9 Scalp BT treatment using the Freiburg flap for a KC postsurgical tumor bed (in red) (**a**) and the corresponding dosimetry (**b**). Note the additional catheters placed beyond the edges of the treatment volume to provide additional dwell positions for adequate coverage (**a**) and the 125% isodose being limited to the skin surface (**b**)

Outcomes

While there is limited high-level evidence for traditional RT in the management of KC, there is no level I evidence for HDR-BT. However, several retrospective and prospective studies with excellent results and reasonable follow-up have been reported. Guix et al. described a standardized surface mold technique prospectively utilizing HDR-BT [10]. One hundred and thirty-six patients with KC achieved 5-year local control of 98% with excellent treatment tolerance and no severe early or late complications. Additionally, Kohler-Brock reported 10-year follow-up on diseases of the skin and mucosal membranes using a standardized small surface applicator, achieving 92% local control. No severe late reactions were reported [11]. More recently, Gauden et al. reported data on 200 patients with 236 KC treated with a standardized HDR applicator. With a median follow-up of 66 months, the local control was 98% and cosmesis was good to excellent in 88% of patients [12]. Tormo reported results of a prospective trial with the Valencia applicator. Thirty-three patients with 48 KC received 42 Gy in 6 fractions. Local control was 98% at a median follow-up of 47 months [13]. Brovchuck et al. reported on 751 patients from a single institution who received either a surface mold (225 patients), interstitial BT (518 patients), or both (8 patients) [14]. Over 60% of the patients were stage 2 or greater. With a 36-month median follow-up, local control was 96%. Excellent cosmetic results were described in 79.9% and good in 17.8%. Patel et al. compared matched cohorts of 208 lesions in 188 patients in an eBT group with 208 lesions in 181 patients in a Mohs micrographic surgery (MMS) group [15]. At a mean follow-up of 3.4 years after completion of treatment, 99.5% of the eBT group and 100% of the MMS were free of recurrence in this appropriately selected group of early-stage KC. Cosmesis was rated as excellent or good in 97.6% of the eBT-treated lesions and 95.7% of the MMS-treated lesions [14].

In conclusion, while no prospective randomized trials have been completed, there is a body of evidence supporting the use of skin BT. The ABS and GEC-ESTRO have developed guidelines for clinical and dosimetric planning, appropriate margin delineation, and applicator selection.

References

1. Ghadjar P, Bojaxhiu B, Simcock M, et al. High dose-rate versus low dose-rate brachytherapy for lip cancer. Int J Radiat Oncol Biol Phys. 2012;83(4):1205–12.
2. Lee CT, Lehrer EJ, Aphale A, Lango M, Galloway TJ, Zaorsky NG. Surgical excision, Mohs micrographic surgery, external-beam radiotherapy, or brachytherapy for indolent skin cancer: an international meta-analysis of 58 studies with 21,000 patients. Cancer. 2019;125:3582–94.
3. Ouhib Z, Kasper M, et al. Aspects of dosimetry and clinical practice of skin brachytherapy: The American Brachytherapy Society working group report. Brachytherapy. 2015;14:840.
4. Kasper ME, Chaudhary AA. Novel treatment options for nonmelanoma skin cancer: focus on electronic brachytherapy. Med Devices (Auckl). 2015;8:493–502. https://doi.org/10.2147/MDER.S61585.
5. Shah C, Ouhib Z, Kamrava M, et al. The American brachytherapy society consensus statement for skin brachytherapy. Brachytherapy. 2020;19(4):415–26. https://doi.org/10.1016/j.brachy.2020.04.004.
6. Guinot JL, Rembielak A, Perez-Calatayud J, et. al. GEC-ESTRO ACROP recommendations in skin brachytherapy. Radiother Oncol J Eur Soc Ther Radiol Oncologia. 2018;126:377–85.
7. Broadland DG, Zitelli JA. Surgical margins for excision of primary cutaneous squamous cell carcinoma. J Am Acad Dermatol. 1992;27:241–8.
8. Bezugly A, Rembielak A. The use of high frequency ultrasound in non-melanoma skin cancer. J Contemp Brachytherapy. 2021;13(4):483–91.
9. Likhacheva AO, Devlin PM, et al. Skin surface brachytherapy: a survey of contemporary practice patterns. Brachytherapy. 2016;16(1):223–9.
10. Guix B, Finestres F, Tello J-I, et. al. Treatment of skin carcinomas of the face by high-dose-rate brachytherapy and custom-made surface molds. Int. J Radiat Oncol. 2000;47:95–102.
11. Kohler-Brock A, Pragger W, Pohlmann S, Kunze S. The indications for and results of HDR afterloading therapy in diseases of the skin and mucosa with standardized surface applicators (the Leipzig ® applicator). Strahlenther Onkol. 1999;175:170–4.
12. Gauden R, Pracy M, Avery AM, et al. HDR brachytherapy for superficial non-melanoma skin cancers. J Med Imaging Radiat Oncol. 2013;57(2):212–7.
13. Tormo A, Celada F, Rodriguez S, et al. Non-melanoma skin cancer treated with HDR Valencia applicator: clinical outcomes. J Contemp Brachytherapy. 2014;6:167–72.
14. Brovchuk S, Park SJ, et al. High dose rate skin brachytherapy with interstitial, surface, or a combination of interstitial and surface mold technique. J Contemp Brachytherapy. 2022;14(2):107–14.
15. Patel R, Strimling R, Doggett S, et al. Comparison of electronic brachytherapy and Mohs micrographic surgery for the treatment of early-stage non-melanoma skin cancer: a matched pair cohort study. J Contemp Brachytherapy. 2017;9(4):338–44.

Part IV
Miscellaneous

Chapter 16
Benign Skin Tumors

Kurian Jones Joseph

Radiotherapy (RT) has traditionally been used to treat several benign conditions. In Germany, nonmalignant conditions comprise about 10–30% of all the indications for RT [1]. In general, radiation doses used to treat benign conditions are well below the prescription ranges for malignant tumors and are typically delivered in shorter treatment schedules. The radiobiological basis for the use of RT to treat benign conditions includes the following [2]:

- Anti-inflammatory effect:
  - Radiotherapy reduces endothelial cell-leukocyte interactions, increases the production of anti-inflammatory cytokines and enhances apoptotic cell death.
- Antiproliferative effect:
  - Radiation prevents cellular growth in the irradiated tissue by inhibiting progression of cells through the mitotic cycle
- Immunomodulatory:
  - Radiation suppresses the local autoimmune processes by regulating the lymphocyte antigenic stimulus

Even though RT can be utilized successfully to manage these tumors, there is significant concern about the potential risk of radiation-induced cancers (RICs). Caution is required, especially in children, young adults, and patients receiving radiation to areas at increased secondary cancer risk. Ogawa et al. recommended avoidance of postoperative irradiation of skin over the thyroid, mammary glands,

K. J. Joseph (✉)
Department of Oncology, University of Alberta, Edmonton, AB, Canada

Division of Radiation Oncology, Cross Cancer Institute, Edmonton, AB, Canada
e-mail: kurian.joseph@albertahealthservices.ca

K. J. Joseph et al. (eds.), *Radiotherapy in Skin Cancer*,
https://doi.org/10.1007/978-3-031-44316-9_16

near the gonads, and in patients of the childhood age [3]. Although the absolute risks of RIC may be very low, this risk needs to be discussed in detail with the patients who opt to receive RT.

Keloid Scars

Keloid scars are benign dermal fibroproliferative tumors that typically appear after repeated surgeries, trauma, and dermal injuries. They occur due to abnormal fibroblastic activity, increased level of collagen production, and reduced level of fibroblast apoptosis as a part of the wound healing process [4]. Keloids mainly affect the 10- to 30-year age group, occurring in 5–15% of the wounds with a special predilection for darker skin (Fig. 16.1) [5].

Treatment of choice for keloids is surgical excision, which carries a recurrence rate of more than 50% [4]. Complete removal of the proliferating core is the key to minimize or prevent regrowth. Intralesional steroid injection and cryotherapy are the other primary treatment options to reduce the risk of recurrence.

Adjuvant RT is one of the most effective treatments for keloid. RT reduces the risk of recurrence to about 10–20% and can be highly beneficial in cases of scar inoperability [6]. Hence, a combination of surgery and adjuvant RT could be an optimal treatment regimen for keloids. The evidence to use RT as monotherapy is limited. Ogawa et al. reported that primary RT can immediately reduce the pain and itchiness, while reduction in size and color of the keloids may take months [7].

Keloid fibroblast cells proliferate rapidly with a multiplication time of 25.9 h, while the same time for normal fibroblasts is 43.5 h [8]. Kal et al. reported that the shorter proliferation time radiobiologically favors delivery of RT by preventing the proliferation of rapidly multiplying cells and inducing cellular apoptosis, thereby

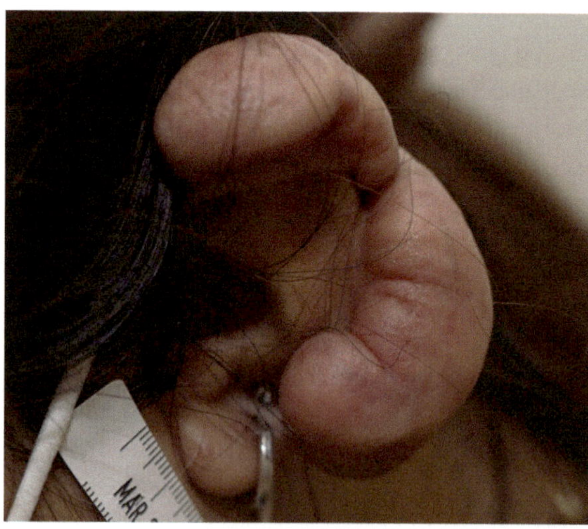

Fig. 16.1 The picture shows left pinna of a 23-year-old woman presenting with keloid scar involving the entire ear lobe. The patient was treated with surgical excision followed by adjuvant RT

reducing the recurrence rates [9]. Due to the active repopulation of fibroblast cells post-surgery, adjuvant RT should be initiated within a shorter time span (ideally within 72 h) to obtain better outcomes. Typically, postoperative RT is delivered within 24 h of surgery for optimal antiproliferative effect [1].

Treatment Planning

External beam radiotherapy (EBRT) and/or brachytherapy are effective to prevent keloid formation. Common EBRT techniques include superficial or orthovoltage RT and electrons. Megavoltage photons are generally not used. The superficial and orthovoltage energy range of 50–200 kV is used to treat most of the keloids. Electron beam energies in the range of 4–10 MeV are most often chosen for large scars. Both low-dose-rate (LDR) and high-dose-rate (HDR) brachytherapy are also considered safe and effective adjuvant treatments for keloids. Surface brachytherapy has been widely used to treat keloids because of its noninvasiveness and low adverse effects.

Target Volume

The target volume includes surgical bed with a small margin of 0.5–1 cm. The field borders for electron beams should include 1–1.5 cm of normal skin around the surgical scar because the radiation doses at the boundary decrease significantly for electron fields. The treatment fields are designed with custom lead cutouts to minimize scatter radiation to normal tissues.

Dose

Bijlard et al. recommended a lower biologically equivalent dose (BED) of >20 Gy for adequate local control [10]. Systematic review by Kal et al. recommended BED values of ≥30 Gy (Fig. 16.2a, b) that would significantly reduce the recurrence rate ≤10% with minimal morbidity [9]. Keloids respond like late-reacting tissues with a relatively low a/b ratio (mean, 2), and hence, hypofractionation is the best approach [4].

Recurrence rate is lower following adjuvant RT in areas without stretch tension such as earlobes, face, and head and neck, whereas in high-tension areas such as anterior chest wall, scapular region, limbs, and trunk, recurrence rates are higher [4]. Hence, different RT dose schedules have been recommended depending on the location of the lesion and the risk of recurrence [8].

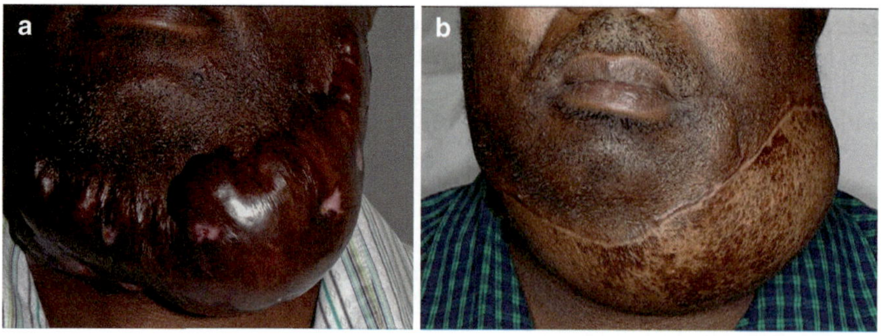

Fig. 16.2 (**a**) shows the picture of a 30-year-old male who presented with an extensive keloid scar of the chin with extension to the neck. The patient underwent wide local excision and skin grafting followed by adjuvant EBRT to a dose of 30 Gy in 15 fractions. Patient shows no evidence of recurrence after 10 years (**b**)

Given the different susceptibility of various body sites to recurrence, a body-site-specific post-op EBRT regimen is recommended [7]. Common fractionation schedules for EBRT are:

- 9–10 Gy in a single fraction 24–48 h after surgery for sites at lower risk of recurrence (e.g., earlobe) with reported local control rates >87%
- 18 Gy in 3 fractions over 3 days for sites at higher risk of recurrence (e.g., anterior chest wall, scapular region, and suprapubic region) with reported local control rates >90%
- 15–16 Gy in 2–3 fractions over 2 or 3 days for other body sites, including the auricle (but not earlobe)

Other recommended RT regimens [4] include:

- 20 Gy/4–5 fractions over 4–5 days for keloids involving the anterior chest, scapula, and upper pubic region; reported control rates >90%
- 10 Gy/2 fractions for the earlobe
- 15 Gy/3 fractions for other sites

Brachytherapy is reported to be more effective than EBRT. The recommended high-dose-rate fractionation schedules [11] are:

- 15–18 Gy /3 fractions over 3 days
- 12 Gy/2 fractions over 2 days

Treatment-related Side Effects

RT is well tolerated with very low risk of complications. The common acute side effects are [4]:

- Erythema
- Wound dehiscence
- Infection
- Desquamation

Chronic complications mainly include skin color changes (hyperpigmentation or hypopigmentation), telangiectasia, xerosis, and skin fibrosis.

Outcomes

Risk of keloid recurrence after adjuvant RT varies from 10 to 20% (Fig. 16.3a, b). The predictors of local recurrence post-RT are:

1. Timing of adjuvant RT—recurrence risk increases with more than 24-h delay in starting RT after surgery
2. Keloid length ≥5 cm
3. Radiation doses with a lower BED <20 Gy

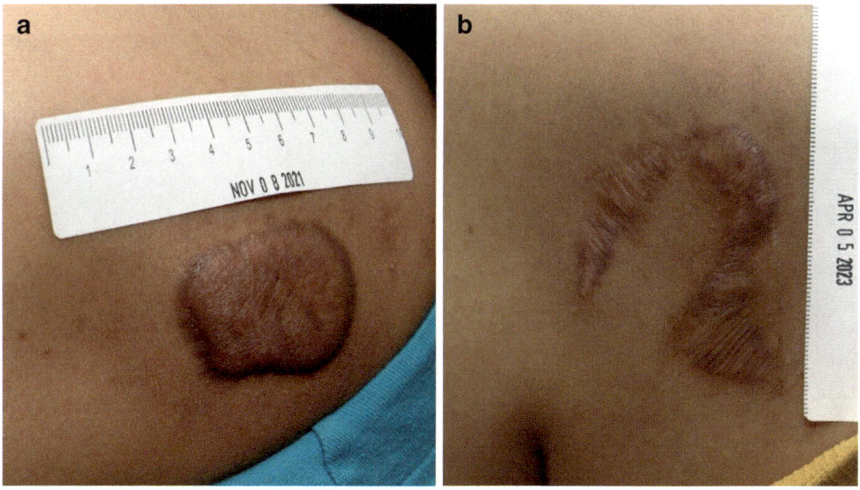

Fig. 16.3 (**a**) A 40-year-old presented with keloid scar of the scapular lesion. The patient was treated with wide excision followed by RT started within 24 h of surgery. Patient received a dose of 15 Gy in 5 fractions (BED = 19.5) using 9 MeV electrons. (**b**) Patient presented with recurrence after 2 years, probably due to the inadequate dose of radiation delivered

Keratoacanthoma

Keratoacanthomas (KAs) are benign skin tumors with majority growing rapidly over weeks and difficult in separating them from well-differentiated squamous cell carcinomas (SCC) of the skin both clinically and pathologically. KAs are most often seen in the middle-aged and elderly patients with long-time ultraviolet light exposure. Lesions are typically found in sun-exposed regions of the body such as scalp, nose, and cheek. KAs are associated with specific disorders like Muir–Torre syndrome, xeroderma pigmentosum, and florid cutaneous papillomatosis [12].

Clinically, KAs present as umbilicated lesions with a central keratin plug (Fig. 16.4a, b).

KAs can be solitary or may present as multiple lesions. In general, KAs initially present as a small red papule with occasional itching and then rapidly grow in about 4–8 weeks to become a large nodule with a craterlike depression in the center [13].

Typically, KAs are characterized by a triphasic pattern of evolution consisting of proliferative (early), stabilized (well-developed), and regressive (late) phases [14]. KA may undergo spontaneous regression in up to 20% of patients that may cause local tissue destruction leaving a scar, especially when the lesions involve the face [15]. This could cause facial or functional deformity.

The accepted treatment options for KA include surgery, RT, photodynamic therapy, and/or chemotherapy. Surgical resection is the treatment of choice for solitary KA.

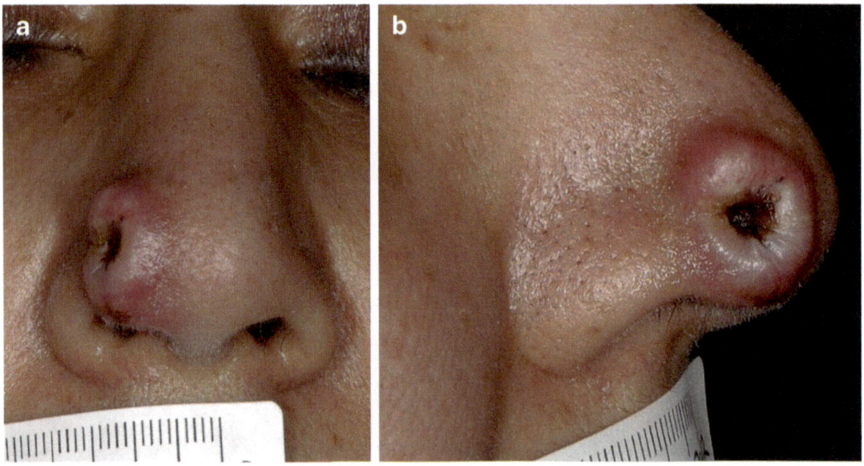

Fig. 16.4 (**a**, **b**) A 50-year-old female presented with KA of the right side of the nose. Clinically, it appeared as a solitary nodular lesion measuring 2 × 2 cm with a central keratin plug. Biopsy from the lesion was reported as most probably KA. The patient was treated with primary RT since the lesion continued to show progression

Indications for Radiotherapy

RT is the preferred treatment for patients who are not good surgical candidates or when surgery can compromise cosmetic or functional outcomes.

Treatment Planning

Target Volume

Treatment can be delivered with either orthovoltage X-rays, electron, or occasionally high-energy photon beams, depending on the location and size of the lesion. The target volume encompasses the primary tumor with an adequate margin. Target volume is usually defined by clinical markup since treatment is commonly delivered by orthovoltage. Usually, a 1–1.5 cm margin is given around the primary tumor which accommodates day-to-day setup variation. If a patient is considered for treatment using electrons or high-energy photons, CT-based planning is recommended.

Dose

There is no consensus on the total dose fractionation regimen and timing of RT.

Hypofractionated schedules are commonly used and are well tolerated. A dose of 25 Gy in 5 fractions over 1 week or its equivalent is recommended for most lesions. However, if the diagnosis is uncertain, a dose schedule similar to an SCC should be prescribed. Current recommendations are:

- 25 Gy in 5 fractions over 1 week
- 40 Gy in 10 fractions over 2 weeks
- 50 Gy in 20 fractions over 4 weeks if the diagnosis (KA vs. SCC) is uncertain

Outcomes

Local recurrence rates following surgery range from 10 to 50% [8]. Figure 16.5a, b shows the response to RT for the patient described in Fig. 16.4, 1 year post-RT.

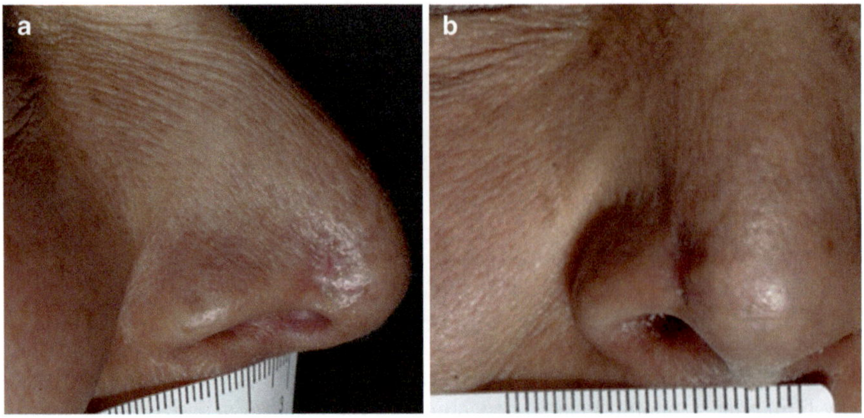

Fig. 16.5 (**a**, **b**) show the response of KA to RT in the patient seen in Fig. 16.4. Patient received 50 Gy in 20 fractions over 4 weeks. The current figure shows no recurrence at 1 year post-RT. Minimal local soft tissue destruction from KA is noticeable

References

1. Seegenschmiedt MH, Micke O, Muecke R. German cooperative group on radiotherapy for non-malignant diseases (GCG-BD). Radiotherapy for non-malignant disorders: state of the art and update of the evidence-based practice guidelines. Br J Radiol. 2015;88(1051):20150080.
2. Torres Royo L, Antelo Redondo G, Árquez Pianetta M, Arenas Prat M. Low-dose radiation therapy for benign pathologies. Rep Pract Oncol Radiother. 2020;25(2):250–4.
3. Ogawa R. The most current algorithms for the treatment and prevention of hypertrophic scars and keloids: a 2020 update of the algorithms published 10 years ago. Plast Reconstr Surg. 2022;149(1):79e–94e.
4. Dong W, Qiu B, Fan F. Adjuvant radiotherapy for keloids. Aesthet Plast Surg. 2022;46(1):489–99.
5. Lee JW, Seol KH. Adjuvant radiotherapy after surgical excision in keloids. Medicina. 2021;57:730.
6. Hoang D, Reznik R, Orgel M, et al. Surgical excision and adjuvant brachytherapy vs external beam radiation for the effective treatment of keloids: 10-year institutional retrospective analysis. Aesthet Surg J. 2017;37:212–25.
7. Ogawa R, Akaishi S, Kuribayashi S, Miyashita T. Keloids and hypertrophic scars can now be cured completely: recent progress in our understanding of the pathogenesis of keloids and hypertrophic scars and the most promising current therapeutic strategy. J Nippon Med Sch. 2016;83(2):46–53. https://doi.org/10.1272/jnms.83.46.
8. Wang W, Zhao J, Zhang C, Zhang W, Jin M, Shao Y. Current advances in the selection of adjuvant radiotherapy regimens for keloid. Front Med (Lausanne). 2022;9:1043840.
9. Kal HB, Veen RE. Biologically effective doses of postoperative radiotherapy in the prevention of keloids dose-effect relationship. Strahlenther Onkol. 2005;181:717–23.
10. Bijlard E, Verduijn GM, Harmeling JX, Dehnad H, Niessen FB, Meijer OWM, Mureau MAM. Optimal high-dose-rate brachytherapy fractionation scheme after keloid excision: a retrospective multicenter comparison of recurrence rates and complications. Int J Radiat Oncol Biol Phys. 2018;100(3):679–86.
11. Nardone V, D'Ippolito E, Grassi R, Sangiovanni A, Gagliardi F, De Marco G, Menditti VS, D'Ambrosio L, Cioce F, Boldrini L, Salvestrini V, Greco C, Desideri I, De Felice F, D'Onofrio

I, Grassi R, Reginelli A, Cappabianca S. Non-oncological radiotherapy: a review of modern approaches. J Pers Med. 2022;12(10):1677.
12. Vergara A, Isarria MJ, Dominguez JD, Gamo R, Rodriguez Peralto JL, Guerra A. Multiple and relapsing keratoacanthomas developing at the edge of the skin grafts site after surgery and after radiotherapy. Dermatol Surg. 2007;33:994–6.
13. Jia X, Ge Y, Wang H. Ma radiotherapy for keratoacanthoma of facial skin: a case report and review of literature. Front Oncol. 2023;12:1032090.
14. Savage JA, Maize JC Sr. Keratoacanthoma clinical behavior: a systematic review. Am J Dermatopathol. 2014;36(5):422–9.
15. Veness MJ. The important role of radiotherapy in patients with non-melanoma skin cancer and other cutaneous entities. J Med Imaging Radiat Oncol. 2008;52(3):278–86.

Chapter 17
Malignant Adnexal Tumors of Skin (MATS)

Aoife Jones Thachuthara and Edward Yu

Malignant adnexal tumors of skin (MATS) are a heterogenous group of rare cutaneous tumors and represent only 0.005% of all skin tumors [1]. Adnexal carcinomas arise from the skin appendages located within the dermis, and there are different histologies based on varying morphologic differentiation toward one or more of the adnexal epithelial structures of the skin, including the pilosebaceous unit, sebaceous glands, apocrine glands, or eccrine glands [2]. Typically, it presents as a solitary dermal nodule, ulcerated or not, located in the head and neck region of an elderly individual (Fig. 17.1). Adnexal tumors are diagnosed by histological evaluation rather than clinically. Histopathological features combined with immunohistochemistry provide a definite diagnosis.

Sebaceous carcinoma is the most frequent cutaneous adnexal malignancy. Common histological types are detailed in Table 17.1.

Over 50% of all lesions occur in the head and neck region, primarily in the Caucasian population [3]. Other common anatomical sites are the upper extremities and trunk. The exact etiology of MATS is unknown. The risk factors reported are increasing age (typically over six decades of life) with ultraviolet light exposure, previous exposure to ionizing radiation, and immunosuppression [1]. Staging of adnexal carcinoma is included in the American Joint Committee on Cancer (AJCC) cutaneous squamous cell carcinoma (SCC) staging [4]. The incidence rates for these tumors have increased by as much as 150% in the last three decades, so it is critical to improve our understanding of these tumors [3]. Tumors are predominantly locally aggressive with a propensity for local invasion and recurrence [1].

A. Jones Thachuthara
Department of Medicine, Beaumont Hospital, Dublin, Ireland

E. Yu (✉)
Department of Oncology and Medical Biophysics, Western University, London, ON, Canada
e-mail: eyu@uwo.ca

K. J. Joseph et al. (eds.), *Radiotherapy in Skin Cancer*,
https://doi.org/10.1007/978-3-031-44316-9_17

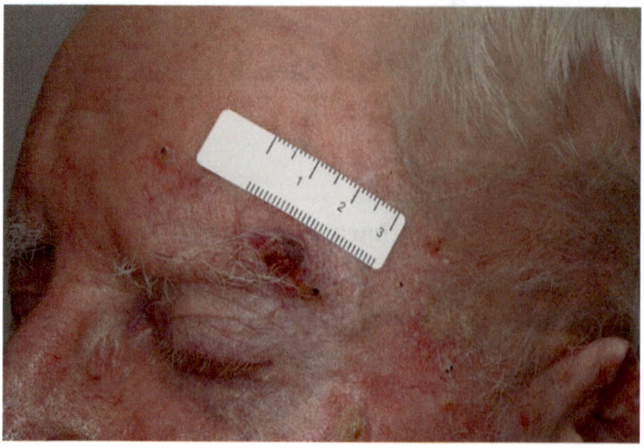

Fig. 17.1 70-Year-old presented with a skin lesion on left forehead of 3-month duration. Biopsy confirmed eccrine ductal carcinoma. Patient underwent wide local excision alone

Table 17.1 Common histological types

Origin	Tumor
Hair follicle	Trichoblastic carcinoma, trichilemmal carcinoma, pilomatrix (matrical) carcinoma, malignant proliferating trichilemmal cyst
Sebaceous gland	Sebaceous carcinoma
Sweat glands	
Eccrine	Porocarcinoma, hidradenocarcinoma, syringomatous carcinoma, microcystic adnexal carcinoma, spiradenocarcinoma, syringoid carcinoma, malignant cylindroma, mucinous carcinoma, adenoid cystic carcinoma
Apocrine	Apocrine carcinoma, syringocystadenocarcinoma
Apocrine eccrine and apocrine (mixed origin)	Malignant mixed tumor of skin
Other sweat gland carcinomas	Eccrine ductal carcinoma, basaloid eccrine carcinoma, squamoid eccrine ductal carcinoma

There is no consensus on the optimal management approach for MATS. Wide local excision or Mohs micrographic surgery (MMS), with at least 1–2 cm excision margins is the mainstay of treatment. Surgical series recommend margins between 3 and 5 cm around the tumor for those who do not undergo MMS, because of widespread infiltration and indistinct boundaries [5, 6].

The potential benefit of routine regional lymph node evaluation is controversial. Locoregional recurrence has been reported in up to 50–60% of lesions treated with surgical excision alone [1, 7]. Sentinel lymph node biopsy can be performed to evaluate the indication for lymph node dissection or selective lymph node dissection could be considered for patients with a high risk of recurrence or locally advanced disease [8].

Indications for Radiotherapy

Currently, there are no consensus guidelines regarding the role of adjuvant radiotherapy for adnexal malignant tumors. In addition, the benefit of adjuvant radiotherapy on locoregional control and overall survival is unclear [9, 10]. Many studies have reported improved locoregional control with postoperative adjuvant radiotherapy in patients with high-risk features; however, most of these studies are small case series or case reports [2]. Although difficult to conclude based on these studies, postoperative adjuvant radiotherapy is still offered with excellent local control in patients with high-risk features (Fig. 17.2).

Patients with one or more high-risk factors are usually recommended to be treated with adjuvant radiotherapy. In general, adjuvant radiotherapy is offered when a patient presents with the one or more of the following high-risk characteristics [11, 12]:

Residual macroscopic disease after surgery
Positive margin
Close pathological margin (<5 mm)
Dermal invasion
Perineural or lymphovascular invasion
Extracapsular extension
High grade

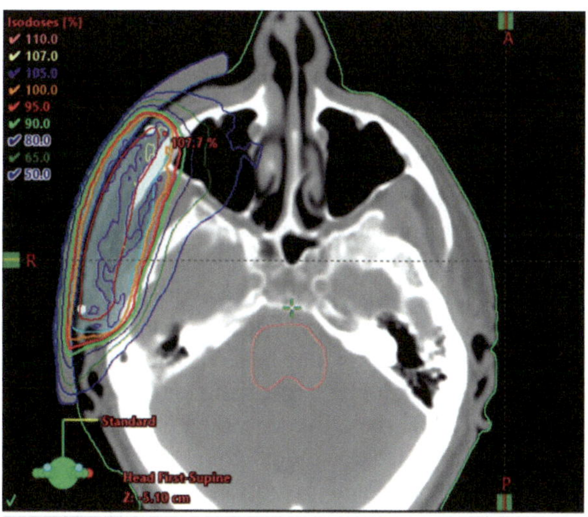

Fig. 17.2 68-Year-old male presented with a small 1 × 1 cm lump on the right temple, and excision biopsy reported as cutaneous squamous cell carcinoma; but re-excision for recurrence within a short time of 3 months confirmed squamoid eccrine carcinoma. The patient underwent wide local excision followed by adjuvant radiotherapy due to associated high-risk features (local recurrence, positive deep margin). No recurrence has occurred at 2 years post-adjuvant radiotherapy

Poorly differentiated
Multifocal disease
Lymph node (LN) involvement
Recurrent disease
T3/T4 disease

Evidence is insufficient to use radiotherapy as monotherapy [9, 10]. However, radiotherapy might be appropriate for patients who are medically inoperable or have tumors or nodal metastases that are surgically unresectable. There are limited reports using definitive radiotherapy for these cancers [13].

Treatment Approach

Adjuvant radiotherapy consists of radiotherapy either to the primary site alone or to the primary site and regional draining lymphatics, which depends on disease stage and is at the discretion of the treating physician. There is no evidence that prophylactic nodal irradiation is required due to the rare event of nodal metastasis (2.1% in the literature) [5]. Patients with high-risk features for locoregional recurrence or with pathologically involved lymph nodes may be offered regional lymph node irradiation.

Treatment Planning

Target Volume

In general, this follows that of treating SCC of the skin. The target volume will include the primary tumor (or surgical site) with or without regional lymph nodes. A margin of 2 cm is drawn around any gross tumor volume (GTV) to define the clinical target volume (CTV) [5, 9, 13]. In case of postoperative adjuvant radiotherapy, the CTV will encompass the surgical bed with an adequate margin, with or without regional lymph nodes. Baxi et al. recommended a 3–5 cm margin around the excision site [5]. The CTV margin may be reduced depending upon the extent of the wide local excision. The planning target volume (PTV) is defined by the addition of a margin of 5–10 mm to the CTV depending on tumor location.

CT planning is recommended for radiotherapy planning. The patient will be lying supine, immobilized if indicated in a custom shell (e.g., head and neck region) and obtaining 3 mm CT slices of the region of interest. The lesion (if present), or excision site, should be marked by lead wire before CT scanning to visualize the lesion in the planning scan. The CTV is defined by adding an isotropic 10–20 mm margin around the GTV or surgical bed. A planning target volume (PTV) margin of 5–10 mm is added around the CTV.

Generally, 3-dimensional conformal radiotherapy (3D-CRT) or intensity-modulated radiotherapy (IMRT) is used for treatment delivery. IMRT may be the preferred technique in terms of a reduced incidence of adverse events compared with 3D-CRT since reduced volume of OARs is exposed to radiation (Fig. 17.3).

Dose

There are a variety of radiation doses and treatment modalities reported to treat MATS in the literature. Excellent locoregional control has been reported in patients who received adjuvant radiotherapy using one of the following fractionation schedules: 50–55 Gy in 20 fractions or 60 Gy in 30 fractions or equivalent (Figs. 17.3 and 17.4).

Local control rates with adjuvant radiotherapy range from 93 to 100% [5, 13–15]. Harari et al. demonstrated complete remissions after radical external beam radiotherapy, using a dose of 70 Gy to primary surgical beds and 50 Gy to regional lymphatic chains [16].

The optimal radiation dose for definitive radiation therapy is still unknown. Some cases treated with a total dose of <65 Gy developed local recurrence [10]. Pugh et al. proposed a dose of 66–70 Gy with standard fractionation or a biologically equivalent dose [15].

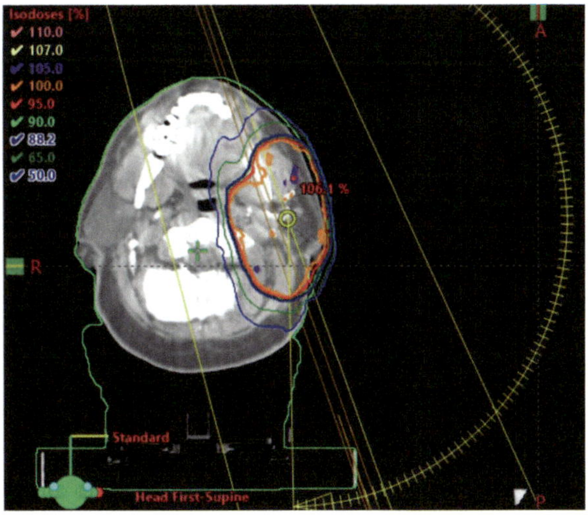

Fig. 17.3 68-Year-old with a 2.1 cm malignant hidradenocarcinoma of the lateral aspect of eye. The patient underwent wide local excision and neck dissection. Patient was staged as pT3N2bM0. Patient received adjuvant radiotherapy with a dose of 50Gy in 20 fractions to the tumor bed and nodal region. Patient is 2 years post-radiotherapy without recurrence

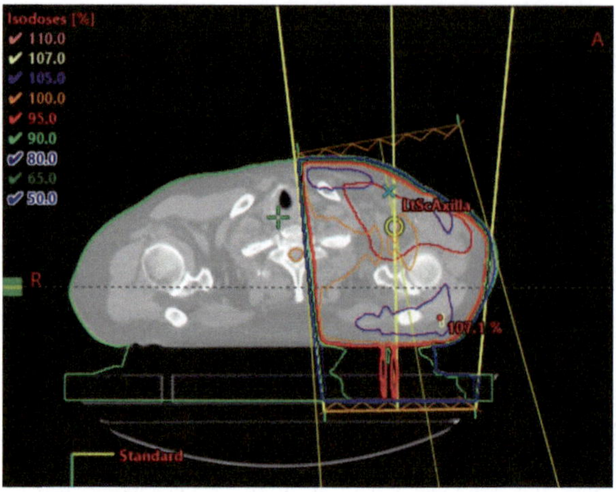

Fig. 17.4 67-Year-old presented with 12 × 16 cm mass in the axilla and underwent radical surgery. Pathology confirmed hidradenocarcinoma. Associated high-risk features were poor differentiation, perineural and lymphovascular invasion, and lymph node involvement. Patient received adjuvant radiotherapy and a dose of 50 Gy in 25 fractions over 5 weeks. Unfortunately, later presented with lung metastases 6 months post-adjuvant radiotherapy

Treatment-related Side Effects

Complications vary according to the primary site and are dose dependent. Common adverse effects for the head and neck region include skin erythema, moist desquamation, hair loss, skin ulceration, mucositis, xerostomia, trismus, or hearing loss. Severe late complications include the risk of soft tissue necrosis, telangiectasia, and second malignancies [11]. However, radiotherapy-induced toxicities are less frequent and better tolerated with modern radiotherapy techniques.

Outcomes

Local recurrence rates following surgery range from 10 to 50% [8]. The mean time for local recurrence was 19.4 (standard deviation: 20.4) months. A 5-year disease-free survival rate of less than 30% has been reported in the literature [17], with 5-year survival rates after surgery in the range of 30–50% [18].

Follow-Up

Patients should be regularly and closely kept in follow-up. At each follow-up, patients should be examined for local recurrence, metastatic spread, and radiation toxicity. If clinically suspected, radiological investigations including CT scan and PET scans may be considered.

References

1. Wang LS, Handorf EA, Wu H, Liu JC, Perlis CS, Galloway TJ. Surgery and adjuvant radiation for high-risk skin adnexal carcinoma of the head and neck. Am J Clin Oncol. 2017;40:429–32.
2. Waqas O, Faisal M, Haider I, Amjad A, Jamshed A, Hussain R. Retrospective study of rare cutaneous malignant adnexal tumors of the head and neck in a tertiary care cancer hospital: a case series. J Med Case Reports. 2017;11:67.
3. Oyasiji T, Tan W, Kane J, et al. Malignant adnexal tumors of the skin: a single institution experience. World J Surg Oncol. 2018;16:99.
4. Edge SB, Compton CC, Fritz AG, Greene FL, Trotti A. AJCC Cancer Staging Manual. 7. New York: Springer-Verlag; 2010.
5. Baxi S, Deb S, Weedon D, Baumann K, Poulsen M. Microcystic adnexal carcinoma of the skin: the role of adjuvant radiotherapy. J Med Imaging Radiat Oncol. 2010;54:477–82.
6. Wong A, Suster S, Nogita, et al. Clear cell eccrine carcinomas of the skin. A clinicopathologic study of nine patients. Cancer. 1994;73:1631–43.
7. Robson A, Green J, Ansari N, et al. Eccrine porocarcinoma (malignant eccrine poroma): a clinicopathologic study of 69 cases. Am J Surg Pathol. 2001;25:710–20.
8. Amel T, Olfa G, Faten H, et al. Metastatic hidradenocarcinoma: Surgery and chemotherapy. N Am J Med Sci. 2009;1:372–4.
9. Owen JL, Kibbi N, Worley B, et al. Sebaceous carcinoma: evidence-based clinical practice guidelines. Lancet Oncol. 2019;20:e699–714.
10. Worley B, Owen JL, Barker CA, et al. Evidence-based clinical practice guidelines for microcystic adnexal carcinoma: informed by a systematic review. JAMA Dermatol. 2019;155:1059–68.
11. Fionda B, Di Stefani A, Lancellotta V, et al. The role of postoperative radiotherapy in eccrine porocarcinoma: a multidisciplinary systematic review. Eur Rev Med Pharmacol Sci. 2022;26:1695–700.
12. Avraham JB, Villines D, Maker VK, August C, Maker AV. Survival after resection of cutaneous adnexal carcinomas with eccrine differentiation: risk factors and trends in outcomes. J Surg Oncol. 2013;108:57–62.
13. Sasamura K, Matsubara D, Kojima M, et al. Intensity modulated radiation therapy for syringomatous carcinoma of the face: a case report. Adv Radiat Oncol. 2019;4:473–7.
14. Guillot B. Unusual cutaneous malignancies: cutaneous adnexal tumours. In: Management of rare adult tumours. Paris: Springer Paris;2009. pp. 471–7.
15. Pugh TJ, Lee NY, Pacheco T, Raben D. Microcystic adnexal carcinoma of the face treated with radiation therapy: a case report and review of the literature. Head Neck. 2012;34:1045–50.
16. Harari PM, Shimm DS, Bangert JL, Cassady JR. The role of radiotherapy in the treatment of malignant sweat gland neoplasms. Cancer. 1990;65:1737–40.
17. Khan BM, Mansha MA, Ali N, Abbasi ANN, Ahmed SM, Qureshi BM, Hidradenocarcinoma: Five years of local and systemic control of a rare sweat gland neoplasm with nodal metatasis Cureus 2018;10(6):e2884.
18. Rehman R, Squires B, Osto M, Quinn T, Kabolizadeh P. Hidradenocarcinoma of the abdominal wall treated with wide surgical excision and adjuvant Radiotherapy. Cureus. 2021;13:e14724.

Index

K. Joseph et al. (eds.), *Radiotherapy in Skin Cancer*,
https://doi.org/10.1007/978-3-031-44316-9

GPSR Compliance

The European Union's (EU) General Product Safety Regulation (GPSR) is a set of rules that requires consumer products to be safe and our obligations to ensure this.

If you have any concerns about our products, you can contact us on ProductSafety@springernature.com

In case Publisher is established outside the EU, the EU authorized representative is:

Springer Nature Customer Service Center GmbH
Europaplatz 3
69115 Heidelberg, Germany

Batch number: 10732090

Printed by Printforce, the Netherlands